Women and Therapy in the Last Third of Life

What is distinct about the last third of life, about women, that makes psychotherapy different? In this diverse collection, the psychological meanings and challenges of the last third of life are explored, as the capacity of the psyche expands, sense of time changes, and some questions take on new vibrance and urgency. Some chapters shine their light on women therapy clients – on their precarious sociocultural predicament in a sexist/ageist time and place, on intrapsychic changes that follow from changing bodies, relationships, involvements and emergent needs of the self. Other chapters enter the largely unexplored territory of changes in the therapy process itself – where some decide against therapy altogether, while others describe a rich revision of familiar elements of therapy, greater authentic presence, a changed standpoint on the power of the therapeutic relationship.

Standing inside the 'last third' and looking back on their own lives, several women psychotherapists offer a rare window into their private experience across time and their perspectives on the challenges and the gifts that they, and other women, may realize in the last third of their lives as they consider who they have become, who they are, and who they can be.

This book was previously published as a special issue of *Women and Therapy*.

Valory Mitchell is Professor at the California School of Professional Psychology at Alliant University, San Francisco. She has been coordinator of the school's Gender Studies Emphasis Area, and Director of its Institute for the Psychology of Women. She is a Fellow at the Rockway Institute, and has a private psychotherapy practice in Berkeley. Since 1978 she has been part of a longitudinal study of the lives and development of 100 women, through UC Berkeley's Institute for Personality and Social Research, with her mentor Ravenna Helson. She is 62, and has a nineteen-year-old daughter in art school.

Women and Therapy in the Last Third of Life

The Long View

Edited by Valory Mitchell

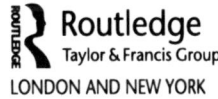

Routledge
Taylor & Francis Group

LONDON AND NEW YORK

First published 2010
by Routledge
2 Park Square, Milton Park, Abingdon, Oxon, OX14 4RN

Simultaneously published in the USA and Canada
by Routledge
270 Madison Avenue, New York, NY 10016

Routledge is an imprint of the Taylor & Francis Group, an informa business

© 2010 Taylor & Francis

Typeset in Garamond by Value Chain, India
Printed and bound in Great Britain by TJI Digital, Padstow, Cornwall

British Library Cataloguing in Publication Data
A catalogue record for this book is available from the British Library

ISBN10: 0-415-56757-2
ISBN13: 978-0-415-56757-2

Contents

Notes on Contributors

ARLENE BERMANN, LCSW, aged 50, received her M.S.W. at the University of California, Berkeley. She provides psychotherapy for individuals and couples and consultation in her private practices in San Francisco and Marin, and as a member of the Psychiatry Department at Kaiser Permanente. She writes and provides trainings on the vulnerability of the therapist in the clinical hour. She has taught courses, lectured or supervised at New College of CA, UCSF/Stanford, and Dominican College. Arlene has a long-standing practice of Buddhist meditation and study which intersects with her contemporary psychoanalytic perspective. She was lay ordained in the Soto Zen tradition in 2006.

AMITY PIERCE BUXTON, aged 79, received her Ph.D. from Teachers College/Faculty Philosophy, Columbia University. She taught every grade from pre-school through graduate school (except junior high years). She helped pioneer the U.S. teachers' center movement and directed two teachers' centers, while writing and giving workshops on active learning, language and professional development, and alternative evaluation. In 1991, she founded the Straight Spouse Network – an organization that provides peer support and informal counseling, worldwide, for straight spouses and couples in mixed-orientation or trans/non-trans marriages, and their families, and education for the larger community. Since 1986, her research, writing, teaching, and board service have focused on these topics.

HARRIET CURTIS-BOLES, aged 55, is an Associate Professor at the California School of Professional Psychology (CSPP) at Alliant University. She received her Ph.D. in psychology from the University of California, Berkeley. She was trained and practices from a psychodynamic orientation, integrating a cultural focus. In her clinical practice at Mills College, she works with women of all ages and from diverse cultural backgrounds. At CSPP-Alliant, she teaches and supervises student research addressing multicultural awareness, communication and intervention, and clinical practice skills. She consults and provides cultural competence training to social service and clinical training agencies in the San Francisco Area. She has been married for 31 years and has an adult daughter.

YVETTE FLORES, aged 57, received her Ph.D. from the University of California, Berkey. She is a professor of Chicano Studies at the University of California, Davis and is an adjunct professor at the Universidad Nacional Autónoma de Mexico in Mexico City, and at the Universidad Santa Maria la Antigua, in Panama. Her research and publications have focused on health, family communication and intra-family violence in Latino and Mexican families, and on Latina girls negotiating identity. She maintains a private practice of adult, adolescent, family, and marital therapy.

MARY M. GERGEN, aged 70, is Professor Emerita of Psychology and Women's Studies at Penn State University, Brandywine. Her Ph.D. is from Temple University. She is author of *Feminist Reconstructions in Psychology: Narrative, Gender and Performance* (Sage, 2001). With Kenneth Gergen, she is editor of the *Positive Aging Newsletter*, a free electronic journal that advocates aging as a time of generativity and delight. She has published in the areas of aging (especially involving women), social constructionism, narrative psychology, qualitative methods, and performative studies. She is co-founder of Taos Institute, promoting the integration of social constructionism into professional practices.

SANDRAH HENRY, LMFT, aged 55 and a breast cancer survivor, is the co-founder of The Laurel Center psychotherapy and training clinic in San Francisco where she sees individuals and couples, and provides training to interns and staff. She is former co-director of the Women's Mental Health Program at New Leaf, an LGBT mental health clinic in San Francisco. She also consults and lectures on the therapist's use of self, disability and illness, and supervision, from a contemporary psychoanalytic perspective. She trained at the Institute for Contemporary Psychoanalysis North, received her MS at San Francisco State University in rehab counseling (emphasis mental health), and a second MS in Marital and Family Therapy at California State University, Dominguez Hills.

JUDITH V. JORDAN is director of the Jean Baker Miller Training Institute at the Wellesley Center For Women, and assistant professor of psychiatry at Harvard Medical School. She received her Ph.D. from Harvard. For the last twenty years, she has worked with colleagues at the Stone Center to create and develop a relational-cultural model of human development. She is author of over forty Stone Center Works in Progress, twenty-five chapters, and has co-authored three books, including *Women's Growth in Connection*. She received the Massachusetts Psychology Association's Career Achievement Award and the Feminist Therapy Institute Special Award for contributions to the development of feminist psychology. She is on the editorial board of the *Journal of Clinical Psychology* and the *Journal of Creativity and Mental Health*.

EMILY LOEB, Ph.D., aged 68, was trained at Columbia University and the Albert Einstein Medical Center in New York. A member of the faculty at the Wright Institute, she is also on the teaching and supervising faculty of The Psychotherapy Institute. Dr. Loeb has written for *The Psychotherapy Institute* journal and NCSPP's journal *Fort Da*. She was first licensed in California in 1976 and has maintained a private practice in the Bay Area for 32 years. Dr. Loeb sees adults in long-term therapy and is particularly interested in working with women who are also tackling time-of-life issues.

LAURA MASON, aged 59, received her Ph.D. in psychology from the University of California, Berkeley. Since 1990, she has been Associate Director of the U.C. Berkeley Psychology Clinic where she oversees the practicum level clinical training of Ph.D. candidates. She also maintains a private practice of psychotherapy, specializing in serving under-served populations who experience moderate to severe psychological distress. Her clinical work is informed by a Jungian and psychodynamic perspective; she has recently added cognitive-behavioral and dialectical behavioral therapy techniques. Currently she serves on the Alameda County Board of Mental Health, and is treasurer of the African Immigrants Social and Cultural Services, a non-profit organization.

VALORY MITCHELL, aged 62, received her Ph.D. in psychology from the University of California, Berkeley. She is a professor of psychology at the California School of Professional Psychology at Alliant University, San Francisco Bay campus, and a fellow at the Rockway Institute of LGBT Studies. Her publications focus on women's psychological development across the adult years, and on lesbian couples and planned two-mother families. She maintains a private practice of psychotherapy with individuals and couples from the teen-age years through late adulthood. Her work is informed by a feminist lifespan developmental psychodynamic perspective. She lives with her partner of ten years and has a daughter in art school in Vancouver, Canada.

HELENE MOGLEN, aged 72, received her Ph.D. in English Literature from Yale University and is Professor Emerita of Literature at the University of California, Santa Cruz. She has written on feminist, cultural and pychoanalytic theory, and on literacy, education and the English novel. Among her book publications are *The Trauma of Gender: A Feminist Theory of the English Novel* and *Charlotte Bronte, The Self Conceived*. With Nancy Chen, she edited *Bodies in the Making: Transgressions and Transformations*, and with Elizabeth Abel and Barbara Chrisian, *Female Subjects in Black and White: Race Psychoanalysis, Feminism*.

SHEILA NAMIR, aged 56, received a Ph.D. in psychology from the University of California, Berkeley, and a Ph.D. in psychoanalysis from the Southern California Psychoanalytic Institute. She was a training and supervising analyst at the Institute of Contemporary Psychoanalysis in Los Angeles and is a clinical psychologist and psychoanalyst practicing in Santa Cruz, California. She was on the faculties of UCLA Medical School, California School of Professional Psychology, and the Southern California Psychoanalytic Institute in Los Angeles. She has published in the areas of psychosocial aspects of AIDS and cancer, medical psychology, trauma and feminist psychoanalysis.

SARALIE PENNINGTON, aged 65, has had a private practice in San Francisco for over 35 years treating adolescents to older adults. She coordinated family, children and queer youth services at Operation Concern/New Leaf, a psychotherapy clinic for the GLBT community, for 23 years. She received her MSW from University of Pittsburgh. Currently teaching at San Francisco State University's School of Social Work, where she began teaching in 1973 in the first wave of Women's Studies, and is considered a "Grandmother" of Feminist Therapy. She is on the Board of Sanville Institute and Open House, a housing/services organization for the GLBT community. She founded Straights For Gay Rights in 1977 and continues as its Chair. She is married and the mother of a 38-year-old daughter, Daria.

SUSAN SANDS, aged 62, has been a clinical psychologist in private practice in Berkeley, CA, for 28 years. She received her Ph.D. in psychology from the University of California, Berkeley. She is currently on the faculty of the Psychoanalytic Institute of Northern California (PINC), an Assistant Clinical Professor, Department of Psychology, UC-Berkeley, and has taught frequently for the Northern California Society for Psychoanalytic Psychology (NCSPP). She was formerly a psychologist in the Eating Disorders Clinic, Department of Psychiatry and Behavioral Medicine, Stanford Medical School. Dr. Sands has presented and published in the areas of eating disorders, trauma and dissociation, and self psychology.

Foreword: The Long View

VALORY MITCHELL

California School of Professional Psychology–Alliant University,
San Francisco, California

The theme of this book—women doing therapy in the last third of life—
suggests that there is something distinct about that time of life, and something distinct about women, something that makes doing therapy different.
But what?

One difference is the sweep of the therapist's personal and professional
experience. Standing inside the "last third" and looking back on her own life,
each of the "autobiographical authors" (Buxton, Curtis-Boles, Flores, Jordan)
in this volume recognizes that she has a view backward some 50–60 to 70
years. Similarly, those taking stock of how the therapy process has changed
for them (Bermann, Loeb, Mason, Pennington, Sands) seem almost to be
looking back through a photo album of "old school" practices, some that
have stood the test of time, and others that are outmoded, discarded now.

Informed by the early feminist recognition that none of us is "objective,"
these authors have spent many years aware of their personal and cultural
contexts and how these situate them and affect their work. Now, they add
an age-linked identity to the other intersecting dimensions that have created
the standpoint from which they take perspective. This recognition parallels
Greene's (2003) understanding of women's development, in which she says
"time [is] a conceptual linchpin for understanding development. Time is
central to both our being and becoming" (p. 15).

Intriguingly, many of the changes that these therapists have observed and
described are manifestations of achievements that lifespan developmental theorists might expect to come with time. For example, the style and concerns that
characterize their therapy process today are similar to the style and concerns of
people who have, across their lifetimes, managed to expand the ego—the syn-
thetic function of the psyche—toward its full potential (Loevinger, 1976).

The desire to help others and to leave a better world for future generations, Erik Erikson's (1960) concept of "generativity," is inherent in the

psychotherapeutic endeavor. But, in this last third of life, it takes on many of the characteristics of Erikson's final stage: ego integrity. Embodying this sense of integrity, several authors have experienced a radical acceptance of the person they've become and the life they've led (Curtis-Boles, Flores, Mason). Another component of ego integrity is the recognition of our own transience, without a sense that death is to be feared. This quality is reflected in the work of those authors who can and do bring death into their work and their planning and do not need to deny its presence (Sands, Henry). The person who has attained integrity is buoyed by a sense of some greater order and resonates with that sense across time, culture, and generations. At the same time, they embrace their own slice of historical time and hold to their style and ways of being. Several authors feel deeply connected with cultural values (their own or others') and spiritual experiences and practices that convey this sense of meaning and transcendence. In all, and facing many directions, these authors have acquired the capacity to take in this long view.

WHAT *IS* THE LAST THIRD OF LIFE?

A few authors chose to take up the task of asking a potentially key question: What *is* the last third of life? We can approach this question from many angles.

When is the "last third"? Sands notes that we cannot know the parameters of the last third of our own life until the day our death comes. Still, she acknowledges that there is "less time ahead, more behind," and she considers how that ambiguity of "how much time" changes the psychological landscape. I have presumed, in a sort of rough-and-ready way, that age 60 demarcates entrance to the "last third." Others would disagree. Amity Pierce Buxton, who, at 79, is our oldest author, asked that she write about herself in the "third quarter of life" because she expects to continue into her hundreds, as have her kin.

Whatever comes, though, a central feature of the "last third" is that it is the last. Several authors (Bermann, Henry) have encouraged us to confront this, not only in its spiritual and psychological implications but in its very practical and relational implications for our clients and colleagues.

In the last third, there is more to integrate. In this volume, many ideas about the psychological concerns of the last third of life have been put forward. The psyche may have a different and enlarged capacity to look within and to accept the nonrational (Loeb). The self-concept, too, expands, as the younger self and the aging self stand side by side. There is a changed sense of the passage of time. There is loss, and the need to mourn for those who've died, for physical losses. Some questions seem to take on a vibrance during this phase of life: What is possible now? What is meaningful? What do we make of all this living we've done—our imperfections, what's been left undone, what we've accomplished and achieved, what's emerged in us over time, what is (or isn't) important to us about any of it? And who are we *really*, distinct from what we've done? What will old age be like? And death?

WOMEN IN THE LAST THIRD OF LIFE

Most of the authors in this volume were just entering adulthood as second wave feminism reached its crest in the early 1960s. Like Zucker and Stewart's (2007) sample of women, these authors have felt feminism shape their lives and perspectives in profound and enduring ways. Some (Pennington, Flores) identify themselves as "feminist foremothers," but even among those who do not put it into words, the evidence of a permanent feminist perspective imbues their writing and their practice.

"Scrutiny with a feminist eye has led to the development of a psychology that, for the first time, includes . . . women's diverse experiences . . . how women perceive themselves or others . . . who women are, and especially . . . who and what women can be" (Kaschak, 1992, p. 10). This promise of a psychology that can result from "scrutiny with a feminist eye" is realized throughout this volume. Here are reflections on an array of different experiences of women, now aged 50–79, who have lived through the late 20th and early 21st centuries. They present distinct perspectives on the challenges and the gifts that they, and other women, may realize in the last third of their lives; they consider who they have become, who they are, and who they can be.

THERAPISTS IN THE LAST THIRD OF LIFE

Several authors took the theme of "women doing therapy in the last third of life" to mean that the "women doing therapy" were therapists in the last third of their lives. These authors have courageously reflected on their personal and professional journeys that led them to today. As a result, we readers get a rare and valuable window into the private experience, across time, of professional women doing this unique, complex work. They are a varied lot, and the themes and roads traveled reflect their variation. And yet, when we step back, their stories share patterns of psychological change and dimensions of inner development that they feel have enriched and enlarged their therapy work.

Each of these authors has "ripened" with time. Some say that they are "more themselves" or allow themselves to use more of who they are and what they have personally known to inform their work. Therapists who are members of nondominant cultural groups describe the years of work they've done to integrate their cultural knowledge and identity with the monocultural professional socialization they endured as students and trainees (Curtis-Boles, Flores). Others have recognized the centrality of early life experiences that shaped them, but which, in earlier years, they had needed to deny or avoid (Mason). Many have grappled with the personal and professional consequences of their gendered socialization. For example, Jordan's autobiographical account of her struggles to have a "voice" makes clear the contact between her work as a creator of developmental theory and her own developing self.

Several authors note how their spiritual practice has informed their work. Bermann and Buxton describe different, yet overlapping, belief systems that have deepened their work. Curtis-Boles tells us that she had first to accumulate sufficient confidence and maturity to override the constraints of her university training and allow a place for her spirituality and thus to be more fully herself as a therapist. Other authors (Mason, Flores) recall powerful spiritual experiences that took place outside of the United States and aided them, upon their return, to claim themselves and their knowledge more fully in their therapy practice.

Several feel that they have softened, become "more comfortable with discomfort," questioned parts of their training that asked them to be less flexible or humane. As a result, they've noticed that their clients have less need to protect them, that the work can go more places than it could when they were younger.

Many believe they have become increasingly able to focus on what is really important and let the rest recede to the periphery. They feel more able to see beneath the surface, to take their time, and to be honest. They report that they have expanded some of their ideas about what is possible, and, in other areas, recognized more limits to what is possible. They have revised their ideas about the meaning and relevance of "curing people"; one author (Bermann) wryly describes her recognition that we all have "fantasies of cure," and hers is that continuing to dye her hair will "cure" her of aging. This more nuanced way of thinking about cure, recognized in both herself and her clients, has helped her differentiate the real possibilities from the illusions.

Several authors have given examples of the way their own psychological development and increased maturity has benefited their work. Some describe that they have discovered structures and practices that help them to listen, remind them of a very large perspective on human joy and suffering, and comfort them.

These realizations are consistent, though not identical, with the research on the characteristics of "experienced" or "expert" therapists. Findings show that experienced clinicians differ from less mature practitioners in being more responsive to the different needs of their clients, being less handicapped by their own "bad moods," being more able to improvise, having stronger self-regulating skills and more flexible repertoires, paying more attention to the client (less self-preoccupation), having a more innovative perspective, and being more likely to make technique decisions that are based on the client's need (Norcross, 2002).

As Loeb (in this book) writes:

> Over these four decades, I've learned a great deal about character structure and about conflict, defenses, and intersubjective experience. I've learned a great deal about listening for the unconscious, about transferences, about timing and interpretation. More than any of all the theory and practice, however, I've learned from my own life experiences. I have a deeper sense of the "human condition," more compassion, more confidence in individuals' innate resilience, and definitely a longer perspective on life's course. (pp. 30–31)

Several authors have been concerned with an even longer view. They may express it in a spiritual way, as though today's healing in a psychotherapy contributes something positive to the whole human condition. Recognizing that by the time we have reached our last third of life we have weeded out much of the "debris," some authors find themselves thinking about the legacy they might leave to a future generation of women and therapists. In this last third, the length of the view extends out past the boundaries of our personal deaths. As Buxton (in this book) writes:

> The core questions for me at this juncture of my life are: Of what value is wisdom that comes with age? To whom is it of value—only to the person who has become wise? If the wisdom of age is of value to others, how can one impart it so that it can help those who survive us to create more enriched lives for themselves and help our professional successors to generate more effective counseling practices? (p. 133)

CLIENTS IN THE LAST THIRD OF LIFE

Other authors (Gergen, Loeb, Mitchell) presumed that the "women doing therapy" were therapy clients in the last third of their lives. Some shone their light on the precarious sociocultural predicament of older women in a sexist/ageist time and place (Gergen), who have undoubtedly internalized these prejudices and stereotypes and will use them against ourselves. Others focused on the intrapsychic changes that follow from changing bodies (Loeb, Bermann, Henry), changing relationships (Flores, Namir), changing kinds of involvement in our communities (Buxton), and changing emergent needs of the self (Loeb, Mitchell, Sands). These authors have given us a sort of composite snapshot of our clients, a glimpse of them in their current moment of life, and they have considered their unique concerns, priorities, and ways of being. Another approach has been to consider a cross-time perspective: What has emerged, or developed? What have the years brought?

THERAPY IN THE LAST THIRD OF LIFE

A third group of authors (Pennington, Henry, Sands) focused on the therapy itself, involving both women. Entering this largely unexplored territory, they tell us about how their vision of therapy has changed. Reflecting on their own practice, they see that they have revised their definitions for familiar elements of therapy—the frame and the therapeutic contract, for example. Some (Namir & Moglen) have even questioned whether women—therapists or clients—*should* be doing therapy in this last third of life.

As varied as they are, *all* of these authors share a view that the development of their therapy work has centered on their ability to be increasingly present in the relationship. They say they are more "themselves" (Flores, Curtis-Boles), more honest (Sands), more comfortable (Bermann), less judgmental and demanding of themselves and their clients (Pennington, Buxton), and more focused on their shared humanity (Mason). They couch their views in "Relational/Cultural Theory" (Jordan) or "Intersubjective Theory" (Henry, Loeb), but, however they say it, they tell us about the power, the value, the almost sacred quality of relationship, and their satisfaction and pride in becoming more and more skilled at it. These authors are all women, but would a group of male therapists say the same? Or is this a women's perspective, a feminist standpoint? Carol Gilligan (1982) posited that women's moral judgments were (more often than men's) based in an ethic of care, and that a facet of women's lifespan development was the expansion of the circle of care to include oneself as well as others. She did not call the centrality of this ethic "relational/cultural" or "intersubjective," and yet these sets of ideas are so congenial with each other and so strongly associated with "women's work," inside and beyond psychotherapy.

Jane Loevinger's (1976) lifespan theory focuses on the development of the mind's internal structure. Describing the later stages of development, she speaks of a sense of internal autonomy in which the psyche is neither driven by affect and impulse nor is it captive to super-ego judgments. The therapists writing in this volume recount their experience of the changes in therapy in a way that resonates with these ideas, too; they speak of spaciousness and stillness, with "more room to breathe."

REFERENCES

Erikson, E. (1960). *Childhood and Society.* New York: Norton.

Gilligan, C. (1982). *In a different voice: Psychological theory and women's development.* Cambridge, MA: Harvard University Press.

Greene, S. (2003). *The psychological development of girls and women: Rethinking change in time.* New York: Routledge.

Kaschak, E. (1992). *Engendered lives: A new psychology of women's experience.* New York: Basic Books.

Loevinger, J. (1976). *Ego development.* San Francisco, CA: Jossey-Bass.

Norcross, J. C. (Ed.). (2002). *Psychotherapy relationships that work: Therapist contributions and responsiveness to patient needs.* New York: Oxford University Press.

Zucker, A., & Stewart, A. (2007). Growing up and growing older: Feminism as a context for women's lives. *Psychology of Women Quarterly, 31*(2), 137–146.

Less Time Ahead, More Behind: Being a Psychotherapist in the Last Third of Life

SUSAN H. SANDS

Psychoanalytic Institute of Northern California, San Francisco, California

For those of us in the last third of life, there is less time ahead and more time behind. The greater proximity to death can lead not only to expansions of the self but to a profoundly revelatory lowering of defenses: it can allow us to acknowledge reality in a way not before possible. The recognition that "life is short" leads to a pruning of activities. The accumulation of years behind us increases perspective and offers a greater sense of the whole. We have ever more "ages inside us," allowing empathy with ever more patients of different (actual and internal) ages. We are more pragmatic, self-regulated, integrated, simply human. There is greater freedom from the rules. The psychotherapy profession, by its very nature, encourages these and other emotional transformations through aging.

As I sit in my Berkeley psychotherapy office, my second home, I know that at 62 I am very different than I was when I began doing this work 30 years ago, or, for that matter, 10 or 20 years ago. I am in the last third of my life—although where in that last third is as yet undetermined. Two things are incontrovertibly true of me now as compared to then. I am closer to death and I have lived more; that is, I have less time in front of me and more time behind. It is these two simple facts that I wish to elaborate in what follows.

LESS TIME AHEAD

When death comes may it find you alive.

—African proverb (2005)

My greater proximity to death brings with it a growing awareness of my own mortality and, if I do not run from it, a greater acceptance of it. As I move inexorably closer to death, it becomes harder to deny its inevitability. Calvin Colarusso (1998) writes:

> In late adulthood, the subjectively perceived *distance from death* is for many a more important organizer of subjective time sense than chronological age. As we age, we look towards death, and we look away. Freud ascribes his companions' inability to feel joy in the beauty of the summer scene around them to "a revolt in their minds against mourning." (p. 306)

I too find myself looking at death, then looking away... looking, looking away. In his famous 1973 book, *The Denial of Death*, Ernest Becker (1973) writes that "*consciousness of death* is the primary repression, not sexuality" (p. 96) and argues that the "terror of death" is a primary motivator of human activity:

> The idea of death, the fear of it, haunts the human animal like nothing else: it is a mainspring of human activity—activity designed largely to avoid the fatality of death, to overcome it by denying in some way that it is the final destiny for man. (p. ix)

In our contemporary culture, we are in a veritable frenzy to try to find "solutions" to the "problems" of aging and death—antiaging serums, life extension programs, age reversal cream—so that we can live "happily ever after." In his essay "On Transience," the 59-year-old Freud (1916) exclaims (through the character of "the poet"):

> No! it is impossible that all this loveliness of Nature and Art, of the world of our sensations and of the world outside, will really fade away into nothing. It would be too senseless and too presumptuous to believe it. Somehow or other this loveliness must be able to persist and to escape all the powers of destruction. (p. 303)

The sages agree: the anticipation of death, which informs the later stages of life, leads to a narcissistic crisis. How we respond to this challenge determines in large part how well we will do in the final third. Our various adaptations to this narcissistic crisis, which have been much discussed by psychologists and poets alike, seem to fall into two categories: first, the defenses which include denial, dissociation, sublimation, bitterness, materialism, and realistic attempts to reverse the appearance of aging and/or to prolong life; and, second, the so-called transformations of narcissism, like creativity, generativity, and expansion of the sense of self.

Expansions of Self

It is the expansion of self-experience that interests me most. The most often discussed way of extending the self, explored first by Erik Erikson (1950), is through "generativity," which he defined as "the interest in establishing and guiding the next generation" (p. 231). Erikson makes it clear that we become generative not only through parenthood but also through other forms of altruistic activity and creativity—among which, I would argue, is doing psychotherapy. Heinz Kohut (1966), in his paper on "Forms and Transformations of Narcissism," introduces the idea of "cosmic narcissism." He argues that those who are able to accept "transience" (i.e., having a finite existence) "do so on the strength of a new, expanded, transformed narcissism: a cosmic narcissism which has transcended the bounds of the individual" (p. 268) and which can, as it were, cushion us in later life from the fear of our personal mortality. He also sees the acceptance of transience as an essential part of wisdom, which he views as the crowning human achievement. Kohut leaves this idea of cosmic narcissism frustratingly vague, but he clearly intends his concept to go beyond generativity to an expansion of self that includes the world and that has as its precursor the early primary identity with the mother. Recently, Charles Fisher (2008) has taken up the concept of an expanded sense of self and how it can provide a creative response to the emotional crisis of facing one's mortality. He argues persuasively that such an expanded self, which can include one's intimates and/or extended clan and/or the world at large, constitutes a "new emotional configuration" in which

> self and object partially overlap without confusion or blurring of boundaries. Mutual interests overshadow competing interest—not merely because it is useful to the person to cooperate with others—but because others are taken as being part of oneself, while still remaining themselves.... the other is treated as a valued part of oneself. (p. 17)

It is my belief that we as psychotherapists are privileged to both live and practice an expanded self more than people in most other professions. The very nature of the work we do helps us negotiate, in a number of ways, the narcissistic crises of older age and impending death. For one thing, doing psychotherapy is a powerful form of generativity. I can feel a great deal of investment in and attachment to my patients as well as pride in their accomplishments—at the same time that my professional training hopefully dissuades and protects me from unhealthy narcissistic investment and overidentification. I do, in certain ways, take my patients into me, and I do in some ways live through them. Moreover, my long years of training and experience in empathy and containment allows and encourages me to both enter into the worlds of my patients and to receive, "hold," and metabolize their unformulated experience in my very being. More contemporary theory on intersubjectivity gives us further metaphors with which to understand ongoing mutual, reciprocal influence within the analytic dyad—that is, all the ways in which we and our patients interpenetrate, on unconscious as well as conscious levels. Complexity theory, or nonlinear dynamic systems theory, takes us one step further into an expanded self as we imagine ourselves embedded in whole systems and fields of mutual influence, to the point where it is hard to conceptualize any longer where one person or entity ends and another begins.

Seeing Things As They Are

The ideas I have discussed thus far remain in the psychological realm, assuming that an expanded self, however felicitous, is an *adaptation* to a narcissistic crisis. There is, however, another way to approach our fears of death. The greater awareness of death that comes with aging can lead not only to adaptive new defenses (including expansions of self) but, even more importantly, to a profoundly transformative *lowering of defenses*. I suggest that the shedding of the veils that accompanies a true encounter with our own mortality allows us to see into and acknowledge reality in a way that is not before possible. There is a new ability to see things as they are.

If, as Becker (1973) argues, all fears are built around our fears of death, and death anxiety is a central part of all anxiety, then, as we become more comfortable staring death in the face, we become more able to meet head-on the other rudely unsettling challenges of life. Picture, if you will, our defenses against our mortality as a much too large lid, one that covers not only death but all manner of difficult, overwhelming, or intolerable experience. If we can crack the lid on death, we may be more able to see and acknowledge our many other fears, doubts, and regrets. Alongside awareness of death, our other challenges may appear more like blips on the radar screen. If we can confront the enormity of our own personal dissolution, then we are much more able to be with what *is*. We become "sadder but wiser." There is a touch of resignation and of the tragic but, hopefully, not too much depression.

In Buddhist thinking (e.g., Buddhaghosa, 1999), Death is one of the Four Messengers whom Prince Siddhartha (later to become the Buddha) encountered when he first explored the world outside his palace gates. The messengers (which also include aging and sickness) are teachings, harbingers of the reality we all have to face. The awakening of the mind to old age and death occurs when we realize at a gut level that these experiences are actually going to happen to us and not only to those other people. The Buddha sent his followers out to the charnel grounds to contemplate the state and decomposition of the body as the first step toward imagining the state and decomposition of one's own dead body and the awakening of the mind that can ensue. For Buddhists, the meditation on death is the supreme meditation.

We are fortunate as psychotherapists to be able to practice, many hours a day over many years, the containment of difficult emotions and truths, including aging, sickness, and death. With this ongoing practice comes a more profound understanding of the reality of human existence. Hedda Bolgar (2006), a psychoanalyst and political activist, says in a film interview conducted when she was 97 years old:

> I live by one idea now, which is that in analysis we don't try to avoid things, we don't try to hide things. We are committed to uncovering things and dealing with it. And I think that needs to be true of the relationship with the patient and it needs to be true of how you live and it needs to be true in every way.

It is this increasingly open-eyed relationship to life (and death) that can make us more and more useful to our patients. We can become more able to *be* with whatever they bring to us. We are less vulnerable and reactive. Our own defenses are less easily mobilized in reaction to our patients' material. Our empathy can deepen, and our ability to provide containment can become more effective, encompassing, and reliable. If we, as older therapists, are able to stay with our awareness of the inevitability of death and our own finitude and not be carried away into manic defenses, I believe we have lifted a major veil and can better help our patients accept "the way things are." We are not truly alive until we can feel ourselves a part of the ongoing cycle of birth, aging, and death that reveals itself all around us and that is the truth of existence.

> And till thine this deep behest:
> Die to win thy being!
> Art thou but a dreary guest
> Upon earth unseeing.
> —Johann Wolfgang von Goethe (1828)

As we age, moreover, we experience the actual deaths of loved ones. I have recently experienced the once-unthinkable death of my mother. Now, no member of my lineage stands between me and my own death. I have seen friends and mentors die. I have discovered that I can endure these painful experiences and survive. The first time I saw death was at the burning ghats in Varanasi, India. I was 27. Since I had only seen death in movies, I somehow expected the experience to be accompanied by sudden, terrifying organ chords. But there were none. I saw bodies burning and melting and falling apart. There was a horrible stench. But the process was undeniably natural, and I felt great curiosity and excitement and especially relief to actually see death with my own eyes. I knew at that time (and I was right) that I would never again look at death—or life—in the same way and that I myself would never be the same. Similarly, as I watched my mother decline during her final few weeks, I experienced firsthand the revelation of the Hospice movement (2006): death is as natural a process as birth. Death proceeds through predictable stages. Activity slows. There is a turning inward. Bodily processes start shutting down. Need for food and drink decreases. Sleepiness increases. Breathing becomes intermittent and finally stops. Heart rate becomes irregular and finally stops. The body cools.

Truly opening oneself to the reality of death can lead to dramatic changes not only in one's sense of self but also in how one chooses to live one's life. From the Kleinian perspective, our confrontation with death gives us another chance to work through the depressive position (e.g., Jaques, 1965), leading to further relinquishment of unconscious omnipotence. We can become more able to tolerate loss and dependency and to sustain love for the important people in our lives despite their shortcomings and destructive aspects. Even death itself can be held as a good object rather than a persecutory one. All this brings greater serenity and emotional stability.

These and other transformations of the self through the aging process are, of course, not always possible. We may not have the internal resources to allow such psychic transmutations, and our later years may be filled—as Erikson (1950) suggested—not with increasing integrity but with despair. But if we are fortunate, our recognition that the future is circumscribed and that time and energy are limited ("life is short") can lead to a pruning of our activities to include, as is possible, only the most crucial and enjoyable. Freud (1916) writes, "Transience value is scarcity value in time. Limitation in the possibility of an enjoyment raises the value of the enjoyment" (p. 304).

As we increasingly acknowledge "scarcity value in time," we come to know that there is limited time for our patients as well as for us. With my patients, I have more of a sense of cutting to the chase. Why wait? I myself live closer to what is important and valuable to me. The essential question beckons: what am I called to do in the time that remains?

MORE TIME BEHIND

Only at the end, can one see what it's all about.

—Margaret Atwood (year unknown)

I have been considering the impact of living in a subjective universe in which there are many fewer years ahead of me than behind and in which the closeness of death and the shortness of time are constant companions. I would now like to turn my gaze backward to the years behind me. What do I find? A huge accretion of experience. As I continue to move inexorably through the unique arc of my particular life, there is more and more to look back on. More and more of the lifecycle opens out behind me. As I see the endless repetitions of my own behavior patterns and those of humankind-at-large, it is harder and harder not to notice and take stock. I have a greater sense of the whole. I recognize patterns. I gain "perspective."

"Only at the end, can one see what it's all about," asserts Margaret Atwood (year unknown). in an interview on the novel-writing process. Similarly, as I advance toward my own end, I can almost see my own life as a story with by now well-developed themes, style, "voice," and characters—a story that I am continuing to write and revise, adding new themes and characters and stumbling on surprise plot twists and unexpected character development. As the years pile up behind me, the essence of my life—with its unique contours, textures and hues—comes increasingly into focus, like a photographic image emerging from the developing bath. Parenthetically, I find a parallel in my own writing: I have come to expect that I will not really understand my own papers until years after writing them.

As I age, I am aware of more and more ages inside me. I contain and am constituted by all the ages that I have lived, and I can experience them simultaneously within me, with their different needs, feelings, quirks, abilities, vulnerabilities, behaviors, and preferences, and I can feel the synergy of their ongoing negotiations, struggles, and collaborations. This knowledge offers a tremendous advantage in doing psychotherapy, as in life. Our awareness of having ever more different-aged selves within us allows us to better empathize with and identify with ever more patients of all different ages—and with all of their different internal ages—as well as with the parents, children, and all the other people in our patients' lives. The more parts of us that we have available—and of course I don't just mean ages—the more we can find analogies between ourselves and others and the many, deep streams of connection.

"Simply Human"

As I get older, there is the deepening understanding that "life is hard." This sobering realization allows me to more easily resonate with the troubles of others with a sense of shared humanity and less sense of distance or separation or (in clinical terms) pathologizing. We are all brothers and sisters in this dark night. The gradual accretion of experience and understanding over the lifespan can give us more compassion, which Buddhist psychology understands as the trembling of the heart in the face of suffering. Compassion, if we are fortunate, flowers as we age. With my patients, I find myself referring to Harry Stack Sullivan's (1947) famous comment, "We are all much more simply human than otherwise" (p. 7). I have also found myself saying something (I don't know where I got it) about how we are not perfect, but perfectly human. These truths are so simply and profoundly comforting. Why withhold them?

Accordingly, I allow myself more freedom to make "simply human" interventions. Alison, a 65-year-old professional woman who lives alone, was speaking one day about her fear of feeling terribly lonely over the holidays. "I'll always be lonely. ... I've gotten nowhere in therapy," she cried. "I'm too wounded." After some moments of silence, I simply said to her, "You know, I think that practically everyone who lives alone has trouble over the holidays." The comfort my comment provided was palpable, and it helped rather than hindered her in going on to explore her own particular feelings around these holidays and holidays in general.

My greater comfort with being simply human as a therapist also allows me to show my true feelings with more spontaneity—grief, joy, shock, whatever I am experiencing. My language is also more matter-of-fact, "regular." I am more likely to share a fantasy arising from nowhere when I think it may shed light on the patient's material. I am more likely to say, when the particular situation calls for it, "I would feel that way too." As an older person, I feel more connected to all living things—animals and plants, as well as people—and less interested in the products of "society," with the exception of the arts, which grow ever more precious. Relationships with others are now of utmost importance, and this, as a psychotherapist, is my privileged focus day after day after day.

Pragmatism

As a therapist in the last third of life, I am also more pragmatic. I try to do what "works" rather than what is deemed appropriate according to contemporary psychoanalytic technique or fashion. There is greater freedom from the rules. Again, I think of my work with Alison, who spent much of her time feeling painfully isolated and lonely. When she was separated from me over weekends or vacations, she would, in her words, "spiral downward." While some success was made over the first two years of treatment, her internal life did not really begin to shift until we modified our treatment structure in a very significant way. With my encouragement, she began calling me regularly and leaving me messages when she felt an urgent need for connection. Sometimes I would get as many as four messages a day, sometimes none at all for several days. Over time, Alison began to feel a little better and to make use of therapy more. She reported that leaving messages was helping her feel "less empty." She reported feeling that "something was happening inside her" and that it was getting easier to imagine that I could actually keep her in my mind when I was away from her.

How do I feel about her leaving so many messages? Honestly, I feel delighted most of the time. I am relieved to have more contact with Alison because it is "working." It is also important that we have found a way of having more contact that does not overburden me. Her brief messages do not intrude on my life; nothing is expected of me except to listen to the messages when and if I have the time. As a therapeutic couple, *we* feel better because we are more effective. When I told Alison that I too felt better having more contact, my comment reassured her immensely, not only because she had been worried about depleting me but because it countered a lifelong anxiety about being "too much" for those around her.

As the years accumulate behind me, I understand more about the cyclical and contextual nature of all personal and societal problems. As a therapist, I am not so surprised when things appear to be going swimmingly, then suddenly fall to pieces, then, just as inexplicably, resolve themselves into some unforeseen level of integration. A wider perspective reveals the impossibility of accurate diagnosis or prognosis, since all symptoms and problems arise out of the dynamic systems in which they are embedded. A striking example comes from my work with Joe and Frieda. When we began, Frieda described Joe as a narcissistic brute (and it was hard not to agree). When Frieda would come home struggling under a heavy load, Joe would not move a muscle and would act surprised and put out if she asked for help. When she was sick in bed, Joe would refuse to acknowledge her illness or take care of her in any way. Then, one weekend, the couple went to visit Joe's parents for the first time, and, lo and behold, Frieda discovered that Joe's mother is fiercely and pathologically "independent" and that she bristles and becomes insulted by any effort to help her. In a different picture frame, Joe suddenly looks like a different person—that is, like a man trying to be a good son by accommodating to his mother's urgent need to feel autonomous.

Emotional Integration

Research on aging (e.g., Carstensen, 2004) suggests that our emotional stability, optimism, and self-regulation do indeed increase as we get older. These enhanced abilities, which I recognize to certain degrees in myself, are enormously important in our work. As my own emotions have become more stable and consistent over time, I have become a better "container" for my patients' overwhelming emotional experience. Because my worldview is generally optimistic, I can better "hold the hope" for my patients when they are going through a rough patch and have lost a sense of a future for themselves.

As I have learned better self-care, I understand more about how to help my patients with their own self-regulation. I am more clear that my ability to self-regulate is determined only in part by my early experiences of affect attunement or my attachment status—those aspects that have been emphasized in psychodynamic thinking—and that self-regulation is also something I have *learned* over the years through repeated and challenging experiences as well as my own psychoanalytic treatment. Moreover, as my body ages and becomes less resilient and needs more care and attention, I must continually learn anew how to self-regulate according to my particular (and changing) needs. All this has helped me become more adept at helping my patients respect and manage their unique bodily and emotional requirements.

Having so many years behind me, I am more realistic about myself. I know more about my own limitations as well as the limitations of even the best and most loving relationships. In my 20s, I vaguely believed that I should be able to become or achieve anything I wanted. In my 30s, I became more aware of the boundaries imposed by my emotional, intellectual, and physical inheritance and by my upbringing and later life experience. That understanding has only increased with the years, bringing with it, yes, certain disappointments and wistfulness but also, more importantly, a sense of being able to use myself more fully as I *am* rather than as who I might be. I know now that I do best when I go with the river rather than against it. With the wider and clearer perspective of older age, I am if anything more aware of the mistakes and poor choices I have made in the past, and it takes a certain ongoing effort to tolerate, forgive, and integrate these more regrettable aspects of myself. I rely less on manic defenses. I am sadder and wiser, more philosophical and more contemplative. I think less about my role as therapist or professional and more about being me. There is less often a "they" that knows more than I do. I can finally do what I want.

All of the above changes and modifications in sense of self and other, which I have suggested can accompany aging, speak to profound inner transformation. Our internal object world, as well as our external world, changes as we age. As we grow older—if all has gone well enough in our development—our internal objects become less parental and godlike, hence less idealized and less feared. We experience them as more "with" us and more forgiving. The demands of these superego figures become more realistic and based increasingly on who we are rather than who we should be. One might say that there is, in our internal world, less distance between our internal parental objects and our internal selves as we ourselves to a greater and greater extent assume the parental function. The internalized parents with whom we have spent a lifetime—whether they have been robust, weak, loving, hateful, vital, or, in Kleinian terms, "dying" or "dead"— become less powerful in our psyches as we ourselves become parents to ourselves.

Aging and experience, of course, are not the only factors. Psychotherapy is often enormously helpful. And our becoming parents ourselves increases our identification with our own parents, both actual and internalized. When our actual parents die, particularly if their deaths are somewhat timely, anticipated, and mourned, our sense of being parents at the apex of the family pyramid is further enhanced.

THE CLINICAL WORK

And what of the clinical work itself? My work continues to feel, much of the time, like the greatest adventure I could pursue. It combines intimate emotional connection, service to others, intense intellectual stimulation, scientific discovery, artistic creation and, to boot, my own personal development. I feel like I am still growing, as a therapist as well as a human being, as a result of the work. It is a profession in which, as a woman, I can be strong, authoritative, smart, successful, and enterprising as well as nurturing, vulnerable, tender, and loving. How could I ask for more than this?

Of course, there are the downsides. At this age, I sometimes find myself less stimulated or challenged by the work than I was as a newer therapist, and I can get a bit complacent. The best corrective is professional enrichment of some kind—consultation, workshops, reading, writing, teaching—to help keep me at my cutting edge. The isolation of private practice strikes me as even stranger now than when I began; there is something unnatural about sitting in a room behind a closed door all day. As a countermeasure, I try as often as possible to build in lunches with friends or other occasions where I can just blither away without constraint. Moreover, since I am constitutionally a very active person, I find the physical passivity of our work difficult, which I try to remedy with trips to the gym and walks with the dog.

At this moment in my life cycle, despite the falling of the flesh and the clouding of the memory, I am grateful to be an older person, and particularly an older therapist. It is a wonderful profession to grow old in. So many of the things that come with aging that I've discussed—increased awareness of death, expanded sense of self, enhanced ability to "see things as they are," wider perspective, multiple ages "inside," increased self-acceptance, a sense of shared humanity—continue to develop and deepen as a consequence of our uniquely challenging work and to the benefit of my work. I am a much better therapist than I was 10, 20, or 30 years ago. This is undoubtedly why so many of us never stop working and why, at this point, I have no plans to retire. I feel blessed to do what I do.

REFERENCES

African proverb, quoted in Nisker, W. (2005, December). Busy dying. *Common Ground*. Retrieved from http://commongroundmag.com/2005/12/dying0512. html.

Becker, E. (1973). *The denial of death*. New York: Free Press Paperbacks.

Bolgar, H. (2006). Film interview, from *The Beauty of Aging*, Laurie Schur, director/producer, www.beautyofaging.com.

Buddhaghosa (1999). *The path of purification* (Visuddhimagga), tr. Bhikkhu Ñanamoli. Onalaska, WA: Pariyatti Publishing.

Carstensen, L. (2004, October 8). Motivation, emotion and aging. *Lecture at 40th Nobel Conference*, Gustavus Adolphus College, Saint Peter, Minnesota.

Colarusso, C. (1998). A developmental line of time sense: In late adulthood and throughout the life cycle. *Psychoanalytic Study of the Child*, 53, 113–140.

Erikson, E. (1950). *Childhood and society*. New York: WW Norton & Co.

Fisher, C. (Submitted). Reading development backwards: What the second half of life teaches us about psychoanalytic theory and technique. *Journal of the American Psychoanalytic Association*.

Freud, S. (1916). On transience. In J. Strachey (Ed.)., *Standard edition* (vol. 14, pp. 303–307). London: Hogarth Press.

Hospice Foundation of America. (2006). *The dying process: A guide for caregivers*. Washington, DC: Hospice Foundation of America.

Jaques, E. (1965). Death and the mid-life crisis. *International Journal of Psychoanalysis, 46*, 502–514.

Kohut, H. (1966). Forms and transformations of narcissism. *Journal of the American Psychoanalytic Association, 14*, 243–272.

Sullivan, H. S. (1947). *Conceptions of modern psychiatry*. Washington, DC: William Alanson White Psychiatric Foundation.

von Goethe, J. (1828). Quoted in Kohut, H. (1966). Forms and transformations of narcissism. *Journal of the American Psychoanalytic Association, 14*, 243–272.

On Becoming an Elder: An Immigrant Latina Therapist Narrative

YVETTE G. FLORES

Chicana/o Studies Program, University of California–Davis, Davis, California

The journey from student to licensed psychologist, from young adult to seasoned and mature clinician, and, last, to elder in the Latino therapeutic community entails multiple migrations. In this paper, I explore the recurrent patterns and themes of these migrations across boundaries of nations, class, sexualities, and family formations within and outside the therapeutic milieu. Interwoven in the narrative is a questioning of the gender roles and cultural mandates that, as a woman, wife, mother, lover, teacher, and clinician I have had to negotiate and renegotiate. Through a feminist lens, I examine the web of relationships, particularly with my chosen sisters, and the path to reclaim a more whole, integrated, spiritual, and embodied self. Positioned as an elder, I examine how this positionality informs and nuances my teaching and clinical work.

BORDER CROSSINGS: SITUATING THE WRITER

I am a clinician, a psychotherapist, and an academic. I teach, do research, and write. Above all, however, I am a transnational migrant, a woman who crosses borders. My first migration occurred before I was one year old. I have no recollection of it; however, the impact of that move from one small Central American country to another shaped the way my parents related to each other, how they raised me, and (invisibly for many years) the way I made life decisions.

The salient themes of my life—attachments (or lack of them), commitments to social justice, the search for "home," the desire to heal sadness and *desarraigo* (lack of rootedness)—emerged from historical legacies of earlier migrants: the French great-grandfather who left France to help build the Panama Canal, the Chinese great-grandfather who left Canton to build the railroads in Costa Rica. These men partnered with *mestizas* (indigenous and African women and daughters of other diasporic European migrations to the Promised Land of the American continent). My parents, offspring of those complicated unions, sought in each other comfort for their own lack of place and belonging. Given the complex racial politics of Latin America, both of my parents thought of themselves as white, and they erased (or hid) their illegitimate and "colored" ancestries.

Given the pain endured in their childhoods, they tried to create a safe haven for my childhood. However, neither could fully give their love. My father spent his life pulled between invisible loyalties to his families of origin and procreation; my mother spent her life longing for what and whom she did not have, unable to be totally present with my father and me. I inherited these loyalty conflicts and yearnings for wholeness and home.

I have spent my adult life trying to interweave the gender, racial, class, and national identities that I embody, through my research, teaching, and clinical work. These also became dominant themes in my quest for balance in my life. In this paper, I look back on the roads traveled and revisit my multiple migrations in order to examine and make visible how these border crossings influenced and continue to guide my clinical work.

Legacies

Like his grandfather before him, my father left his homeland purportedly to seek a better life. He went from Costa Rica to Panama since there was abundant work for adventurous young men, given the country's strategic Canal and U.S. military presence. However, my father also left because his mother had died the year before and his own father had further broken his heart by almost immediately bringing his young mistress to the family home so she could raise his six orphaned children, of whom my father was the eldest. My father instead left the country and was temporarily cut off from his progenitor. In Panama, he found both work and an older, separated woman with two sons, with whom he formed a union. I was born, like my mother before me, out of wedlock. This was a secret my mother kept until I was in my late 20s and pregnant with my first child.

Both of my parents described an idyllic life in Panama. They both regretted leaving the country, although for different reasons. My father returned to Costa Rica, pulled by his loyalty to his father. My mother, following the mandates of her gender and cultural script, followed him, leaving behind her two young adult sons. This migration began a chain of subsequent migrations that would repeat the patterns of our genealogy— disconnection, grief, and psychological homelessness.

Migrations

While I was still a baby, my parents left my native Panama and moved to San José, Costa Rica, my father's homeland.[1] I grew up in a bicultural home. My mother's Caribbean Spanish textured my dreams and my early love of books; my father's slower-paced inflections explained the outside world. My father's position as *el primogenito* (first born male) ensured my rightful place within the patriarchal structure of his large extended family. My mother, the foreigner, whispered in my ear that we came from a different and better place. She reminded me that we did not belong in my father's country, the only homeland I had known since infancy. My mother's quiet rebellion against the patriarchal order "othered" me. I was not to be a *tica* (citizen of Costa Rica). We came from a land of *palmeras, mar, y sol* (palm trees, sea, and sun). I was *Panameña*, my mother insisted. Our yearly visits to her (my?) native land suggested otherwise. My *tico* accent was the subject of jokes and loving chiding. My Panamanian relatives tried to "panamenize" me every summer for 12 years. Upon my return to Costa Rica and my schoolmates every new academic year, the Panamanian inflections that had infused my Spanish were once again the subject of ridicule. So I learned to shift accents and adopt different inflections with every border crossed. This is something I still do, unconsciously. Within days, and sometimes only hours, I begin to match the accents of those whose homeland I am visiting.

I began to come of age in San Jose, Costa Rica, in a neighborhood prophetically named Barrio Mexico. I learned early to camouflage, to adapt, to be a chameleon, to be a *tica-panameña* or a *panameña-tica* depending on the country in which I found myself. From a developmental perspective, I was prime to integrate these identities, when Father decided to migrate once again.

The promise of economic advancement, coupled with the need to escape an oppressive family situation and the consequences of his infidelity led my father to make the pilgrimage from his native Costa Rica to Southern California in 1964. For my mother, however, this second transnational migration took her further away from her homeland and her sons.

---

[1]See Flores-Ortiz (2000) for an elaboration of this migration. *Transnational* implies the ability to remain connected to multiple lands and identities without undue conflict. Inherent in this experience is the freedom to be (and feel) whole regardless of geographical location.

Adolescence in the United States

My first conscious migration occurred when I was 13, when Father announced, by way of a question, that we were moving to the United States, *"Hija, que te parece si nos vamos a vivir a Estados Unidos?"* (Daughter, what would you think if we go to live in the United States?) I felt the earth open up beneath my feet, but not enough to swallow me. Years later, reading Tomás Rivera's (1987) book *Y No Se Lo Tragó la Tierra* (*And the Earth Did Not Swallow Me*), I found the words to describe my experience. Within the rules of our family, Father's question was rhetorical; I already knew that a man's word was the law. My father had decided we would migrate. There was nothing more to be said. Within a few weeks he was gone. My mother and I were left behind to tie up loose ends. That was women's work—to prepare for the migration, to say good-bye, to grieve. For nine months we prepared, Mother and I. She gave away our few possessions and packed her treasures, along with her dreams, into an old suitcase. For years I believed the story my parents cocreated: that we left Costa Rica because father wanted *me* to have a better life and attain a good education.

Years later I would learn the other side of that story. However, I would not fully comprehend the decisions my parents made and the forces that influenced those decisions until I became an elder—an *abuelita* (a grandmother), *tita* for short; a senior faculty member—full professor, scholar, and researcher; and a "mature" clinician.

April 11 marks the celebration of the life and death of Juan Santamaria. As a school child in Costa Rica I had celebrated this date as the (more than hundred year) anniversary of the battle of San Jacinto, where our only relative known to be a hero, Juan Santamaria, had died keeping William Walker and his band of United States mercenaries from invading Costa Rica.

On April 11, 1965, Mother and I along with a cousin descended from the skies onto the runway of Los Angeles International Airport. I wondered if Juan Santamaria was somersaulting in his grave. Thus began my journey of adaptation to the United States. Within two days I was enrolled in a large urban middle school. I encountered blatant discrimination for the first time; I was once again an "other," not Mexican, not Puerto Rican, not White, not Black, not Asian, not American. Yet I felt a kinship toward all. I refused to isolate myself within one particular ethnic group. Thus began my life as a woman nonaligned. My school friends were Theresa from China and Elva from Iceland. After school and on weekends I socialized with relatives and family friends from Central America. Shortly after our arrival, my family went to see *West Side Story*. For days I would sing, to my mother's dismay: "I do not want to live in America . . ."

Within months of our arrival, Mother became depressed, and I became the overachiever, the child of immigrants who must succeed, give meaning to the sacrifices of the parents, and actualize their "American Dream" (Falicov, 1998). I learned English in three months and was removed from special courses for "non-English speakers (NES)" and mainstreamed, after attending summer school. I left my NES friends behind as I had left friends behind when leaving Costa Rica.

I continued to leave my friends, as my parents fled from South Central Los Angeles after the summer of 1965 and moved to a better school district in the San Fernando Valley, after my ninth grade graduation. I found myself to be one of the few Latinas in the college-bound track of my high school. My friends at school were Jewish boys and girls. I continued to live a United Statian existence at school and a Latina immigrant life at home.

During my adolescent years, I learned to navigate the changes in meaning systems that occurred after each migration (Falicov, 1998). I learned to create a social and psychological space that provided continuity with the countries and relations left behind. My connection to my language and culture was a protective factor as I faced racism and gender discrimination within and outside of school. Several of my high school teachers called me Maria, Eva, Yvonne—they seemed unable to remember my name. I smiled and answered their questions, internalizing the rage. But others, including an immigrant German Jewish man and a French immigrant woman, nurtured my intellect and affirmed who I was by speaking to me in Spanish. That was our common language, as each taught me her and his respective discipline. So I learned World Literature and French from teachers who also felt they did not belong.

THE EARLY ADULT YEARS: TAKING HOLD AND LETTING GO

My journeys to pursue my education continued up and down the California coast. I continued to leave people behind. In pursuit of the "American Dream" I grew distant from extended family. I failed to notice my parents' aging and increasing needs. I tried to remain loyal to my ethnic/racial/national roots. I became an activist; I fought for social justice and chose clinical psychology as a field to fill the service gaps I saw as a young undergraduate. I married an older, divorced Chicano man with children as an unconscious political act to remain loyal to my father's and my nuclear family's working class origins. However, without realizing it, with each professional job I acquired I became middle class. I also became a mother, a commuter to various jobs, and a migrant with a PhD who needed to hold two jobs to make ends meet and keep my children in private school in an effort to spare them (or at least attenuate) the racism I had endured during my years of schooling.

Negotiating Identities

During my 20s and 30s, slowly and unconsciously, I wove an identity nuanced by experience and oppositionality. Every barrier I encountered became a challenge I would conquer. I was drawn to psychology by the disorientation and grief my nuclear family experienced as a consequence of multiple migrations. I wanted to be a resource to families in distress. After obtaining my doctorate, I began my life as a therapist and academic, focusing on the pain of addiction, violence, depression, and injustice that plagued immigrant communities. In my own therapy I discovered that my drive to help and heal was fueled by my own invisible loyalties and my multiracial family's own history of despair, resilience, and hope.

But I lived suspended in between nations, loyalties, commitments, and obligations. I was a woman, but I was not free. I was a feminist, but I was bound by traditions and expectations I did not create myself. I married for my mother so she could see her daughter in a wedding gown and cease the whispering behind her back about her daughter who lived in sin. I had become educated for her and for myself. At age 40 I began to live for me.

A Return

My early years as a clinician focused on treating families like mine, who struggled with the sequelae of migration—power imbalances in marriage, underacculturated parents and overacculturated children, injustice in the family. By 1994 I was drained, burned out, and in need of a change in my life. I applied for and won a teaching Fulbright to Panama.

I went home to the land of my birth, where I had not lived in 41 years, and taught family therapy at a Catholic University. Soon thereafter, I was invited to collaborate with feminist activists who were fighting against the social and domestic abuse of women. Through my colleagues, friends, and students I began to regain a more solid identity. As I walked on the streets of Panama, I remembered Mother's stories about her mother, about the violence she endured being married to a good-looking Franco-Panamanian who drank too much and loved too many women (except his wife and daughter). I began to remember the stories told by Mother about our family. My family's history began to come alive just at the time that my mother's history began to recede as a result of dementia (see Flores, 2008).

During my stay in Panama, it became evident to me that, like my ancestors before me, I too could cross borders; I could teach, do research, and practice psychotherapy in Panama as well as in Costa Rica. Moreover, unlike my ancestors, I could return to my homeland and leave it without a permanent good-bye. After half a year I chose to return with my children to the United States rather than stay in Panama, because I felt that my work in the United States was not done. Also I knew that I could go home again, if

I needed to, if I chose to. Panama and Costa Rica were in my heart. I could be in the United States without feeling split, divided, or psychologically homeless (Hardy, 2008). I could live my *Latinidad* in the United States without too much internal conflict (or so I believed).

During the next four years or so, my clinical practice gradually shifted from families to women who were a lot like me: in their mid-40s, established professionals, married or partnered, and beginning to question the meaning of it all. In my own therapy, my healer encouraged me to give more to myself and less to others, to wean the emotional dependency that my status and family position created for too many family members. My clients brought in similar issues. I seemed more successful in facilitating that change in clients than in my own life. So I did what my ancestors had done for generations: I migrated once again.

The Search for a Whole Self

On June 22, 1999, I left behind my life in California to cross another border, to pursue new dreams. I packed lightly, the bare necessities—the anguish of my failing marriage, photos of my children, sage from New Mexico, my husband's last embrace, my favorite books, transitional objects to guide my stay in Mexico.

When the pilot announced that we would descend soon to Mexico City, my heart leapt with joy and anticipation. *Mexico Lindo y Querido. Aqui estoy de nuevo, vengo a caminar por tus calles.* (Beautiful and beloved Mexico. Here I am again. I come here to walk your streets, in search of who I am.) The privilege of my education and the trust of a colleague were bringing me back to Mexico. I would serve as coordinator of the Fogarty Research Program[2] that summer. I would work with three Mexican colleagues and help supervise the work of four graduate students and one newly graduated undergraduate. We were all Latinos, more or less. Over the next three months, we were to do research and learn about Mexico and its people.

Far more than that had brought me there, however. I had fallen in love with the country one year before, when another academic exercise brought me to Mexico City. I walked the city streets, feeling at last that I had come home. I did not understand then why this city of 29 million people filled my heart with joy and made my spirit soar. Perhaps this time, this visit, I would come to understand how a *panameña-tica* felt at last that she belonged in a land that was not her own.

---

[2]The Fogarty Research program, in 1999, focused on creating partnerships between U.S. graduate students and Mexican scholar-researchers. The program's principal investigator was Steven R. Lopez, PhD, then professor of psychology at UCLA. I was program leader and visiting faculty in the summer of 1999.

An uneventful taxi ride, quite a rarity in this maddening city of congested streets and manic drivers, took me to the place I would call home for the next three months. I liked my apartment. It was small, lacking the spaciousness and openness of my home in Berkeley, California. My bedroom window opened onto an open space with willowy trees that swayed with the breeze. It was a recreation area in the midst of a *colonia* (neighborhood). To counter the pollution so rampant in the city, green open spaces were created. Joggers, walkers, and lovers would pass before me in the weeks ahead and fill my hours of solitude. This small humble apartment would become my haven. I had longed for this space, without knowing it. Here, within these walls I would peel away the layers of despair and sorrow and try to find myself, the woman lost in the maze created by loyalty and obligation.

I had become a workaholic over the past 15 years. As my marriage failed, I focused on work and raising my children. I was a good mother, a good daughter. I was a respected scholar and clinician, but I was not a good caretaker of myself. In my little apartment, in this enormous city, I hoped I could find the anonymity that would help me reconnect with my body and my spirit. Here I would be another foreigner, a sojourner, with no ties or connections—except for one, perhaps.

A year earlier I had met a man who reawakened in me desires I had buried under work and obligation. A chance encounter had resulted in an intense, passionate and brief forbidden relationship that would mark the beginning of the end of my marriage. Unlike my father, who had chosen his wife and child over his lover, I had decided to leave both the husband and the lover in order to find me.

Hermanas/Sisters

My friend and colleague Ines Hernandez Avila was in Mexico that summer as well. The Creator takes care of me in this way. My sister was here to help with my transition to Mexico, to this journey of learning I had begun. It was only fitting she be here. She and another friend had initially sent me the announcement of this fellowship and encouraged me to apply. Only six months before, being in Mexico for a summer had seemed only a dream. And now here we were, at the entrance of Teotihuacan.

In Teotihuacan, Ines led our prayers once we arrived, asking for permission to enter the sacred place. How different this experience was to be from the others; I had been there before, the proverbial tourist, exploring, photographing, and while thinking about those who initially inhabited this place not once had I thought about asking them permission to enter.

We climbed the Pyramid of the Moon and prayed for female energy. We prayed to our grandmothers. Atop the pyramid I felt so much sadness I wanted to cry, and a few tears streamed down my face. But I felt good. My thighs hurt but I felt strong as a person, as a woman. Atop the pyramid the gentle breezes reminded me to breathe and carried our prayers upward, toward the blue skies. Nowhere had I seen such blue skies as in this holy site.

The climb and the descent were not as arduous as the first time I visited. I felt stronger physically, and clearly the experience energized me because I had minimal difficulty climbing the Sun Pyramid. Going up, I prayed, as I generally do, for my daughters and granddaughters, sons and other loved ones.

Atop the Sun Pyramid we each prayed for energy, balance, and strength. Then we blessed our things and descended. On the way down, I had an insight. The steps are steep, and there is a section where there is nothing to hold on to. I began to tell myself, "You were once a dancer, agile and strong; you can do this." Suddenly, I realized that my mother had constructed a view of me as a *patiahuada* (a Panamanian expression to describe some-one who is clumsy; literally it means soft-footed); the story being that I was always falling and clumsy, but I am not really that way. I was a dancer. I was not a great dancer, but I had potential. I could do it again. I could be agile, limber, and strong. Then I felt disloyal to Mom and felt sad. But I did want to be in charge of my body again, to inhabit it. A male therapist once told me I did not have a brain; instead he claimed I had a Pentium processor. I took it as a compliment. I had spent years nurturing my brain, but to be a good hea-ler I had had to reconnect to spirit. What about my heart, I wondered? I had chosen a path of service to others. However, I remained somewhat disembo-died and disconnected from myself. With Ines, I began to reconnect to Spirit, to trust my intuition, and to allow myself to be guided into self-healing.

Gender and Power

While in Mexico, issues surrounding national and gender identity became salient for me. The only place where I truly felt Panamanian was there, per-haps because I did not need to explain to people where Panama was or why I had light skin. I preferred not to tell people I was from the United States, despite my 34 years of residence there, because I had never felt United Statian. In terms of my national identity, I am from the place of my birth. In terms of ethnic identity, I think of myself as *pan-Latina, un poquito de aquí y un poquito de allá* (a little bit from here, a little bit from there).

But in Mexico, I was a *mestiza* to my indigenous friends. To them my identity was never an issue. I was not *gringa* (United States), I was not *Mexicana*; I was *mestiza*. I looked European to them. Despite the hospitality of most Mexicans, I could not help but feel like an intruder at times. I did not feel at home with my *mestizo* Mexican colleagues; I was clearly a guest in their country, homes, and institutions.

They generally commented on my "good Spanish." Damn right it was good, I had spent 34 years resisting linguistic assimilation, reading Spanish literature, speaking Spanish at home, in order to remain connected, of all things, to the colonizer's language. Indeed it was ironic. My ethnic identity was connected to a history of colonization. I look like the conqueror but my spirit is aligned with the defeated. In part, I suppose, that is why Mexico was so appealing to me. The contradictions were everywhere. Through my immigrant/tourist/*mestiza* eyes I could see the contradictions and identify with them.

GENDER

My femaleness added to the complexity. Men, both in Mexico and in the United States, generally assume that I am a feminist because I am educated and often travel alone. This assumption sometimes led to heated conversations regarding their ideas about feminism. Also, because of my appearance and accent, it was difficult to guess my ethnic, racial, or national origins. Mexicans often struggled as they tried to "locate" me, as often happened in the United States. A taxi driver one day asked if I was from the *provincias* (central, more rural states of Mexico) or if I was from another country. I hesitated a moment but I told the taxi driver I was from Panama. Others asked me what I did for a living, when I took taxis by myself. When my lover and I took taxis together, I did not exist; the conversations were with him. He gave directions, he negotiated fares, he became the ethnographer on my behalf, and I listened. I listened for their accents, their politics, and their worries. From the private taxi drivers, who dressed well, often spoke English, and had some high school education at least, to the drivers of the dangerous little green VW bugs, I loved listening to men's stories, particularly when they were *not* talking to me. Through my psychologist lenses I wondered how these men survived 12-hour shifts driving in that overcrowded, hurried city. What did they do when they went home? How did they treat the women in their lives? I wondered what they though of me, as I rode alone in their cabs. When I was with a man, they did not need to think about me. I was clearly his *señora* (a term that implies being a wife or partner of a man). I finally surrendered and stopped asking my lover to not refer to me that way. What else could I be, if not his *señora*? It would be improper to refer to me as his lover, and he refused to say I was just a friend (as he felt proprietary rights over me). My preferred descriptor of *compañera* made sense only in progressive circles. But it would not matter really; the assumptions were made. And for me, this was not a battle worth fighting, in Mexico or the States.

While in Mexico, my friend Ines and I often discussed our parallel processes in life. She is from the North, an indigenous and Chicana woman who can cross borders as an *indigena*. I cross borders too, but only as a foreigner. In addition to the question of belonging or not belonging, both Ines and I were beginning to struggle with our age/ing. Seeing the young women who were with us in the Fogarty program, we became aware of how Mexican men perceived us. As tradition dictates, young men asked my permission before asking the young women to dance. I was clearly viewed as the *doña* (the chaperone). Ines and I were not seen as objects of desire—at least not as often as when we were young—and we were expected to act our age. Did I need to act my age? But I did not know how a vibrant 47-year-old was supposed to act.

My visit to Teotihuacan with Ines had a tremendous impact on me. Afterward I felt like crying for days. I could feel the sadness inside me, the desire for connection, and the longing for a love that had been unattainable. I fall in love with men who cannot give, or whose love exacts too high a price. I wanted to be clear about what I do to create distance and thus distinguish it from men's strategies of disconnection. I have seen it in my clinical work with Latino couples, this dance of closeness and disconnection. Can we descendants of multiple diasporas love without so much pain? My parents could not. My first husband and I could not. Would I ever? Would my children?

POWER

During my sojourn in Mexico I became clear about the need to separate my internal process from what I felt about my lover and what was elicited within me by his behavior toward me. I needed to be clear about all of these dimensions in order to speak justly, fairly, and ask for what I wanted. Otherwise, I would lose my power. I could not afford to lose my power. However, I needed to learn to negotiate power from my position as a transnational woman who crossed borders to find herself and to love a man.

At that point in my life I didn't know if I knew how to be in relationship, although my degree and experience suggested that I was "an expert" on the subject. Did I know how to be a *compañera*, other than in the political sense? How does one negotiate equality in the midst of a relationship that is forbidden and nuanced by patriarchal assumptions and expectations? How does one find herself without feeling selfish and self indulgent? My working-class origins and traditional cultural values mandated sacrifice for family. My political views demanded sacrifice for community. My gender socialization intruded into my desire to become whole. I reflected on my women clients and their similar struggles. My compassion grew as I recognized and connected emotionally to the depth of my own pain.

Family, by Blood and by Choice

During my 30s and early 40s, I had distanced myself from extended family in the United States while cultivating an extended network of women who also had histories of diasporic migrations and class struggles and who held feminist views and were strongly committed to social justice. These women had provided me the support I needed to become an academic, to maintain some degree of balance, given my multiple obligations. They were the sisters I did not have, cheerleaders, critics, analysts, and containers for my grief in times of need. Away from them in Mexico, I consciously acknowledged their support over the years.

Likewise, in Mexico I became more cognizant of my parents' role in my professional development. I had been able to become the successful professor and clinician due in large measure to my mother's dedication to my children since they were small. I could travel and write, teach and heal because she and my father provided logistical support and loving presence for my children when I was gone. I did not realize fully their contributions until they both became ill and I had to become their caregiver (Flores, 2008).

My trip to Mexico was cut short as my father became gravelly ill and I had to return home to take over my mother's care and "step up" to the family responsibilities that I had temporarily abandoned (according to my husband and children). My son wrote me an e-mail to inform me that Father was hospitalized and proceeded to state that I "should have waited until my parents died and he and his sister were fully grown" before I started to do what I wanted. My beloved son whom I had raised to be fair, just, and sensitive tried to put me in my cultural familial place, exercising the authority his gender and cultural socialization gave him. I bristled at his statement because it contained a kernel of truth. I needed to face my responsibilities, and take care of me, without running away.

I returned to the United States to enact the culturally mandated roles of dutiful daughter and mother. I took care of my aging parents and my adolescent children but let go of a marriage that no longer worked.

FROM MATURE WOMAN TO ELDER

Nearly 10 years later, as I write this essay, I read my journal entries written in Mexico in 1999. I have grown a lot since then. Indeed, my father's illness and death in 2001 and my mother's waning abilities as a result of dementia forced me into a fully adult role. I had to stop running away to Mexico. I had to embrace my status in the family. As the only legitimate child of my father (the first born in his family), upon his death I became the elder of my generation.

While this "leap toward maturity" was partially in response to my parents' needs, it was due in great measure to my spiritual reawakening in Mexico. I had been in therapy for over 10 years and had worked on many issues, but I still remained very much "in my head," despite my therapist's efforts to help me reconnect to my body. In Mexico I began to pray again. Upon my return, I began to study with an elder, who had told me 20 years before (when we first met) that I was *Pacha Mama* (Mother Earth) and that one day I would hear my song. I did indeed hear my song, while working with a Native American healer. I heard it as she told me I was going to lose my head. I did not quite understand what she meant, but at the level of spirit I fully knew what lay ahead.

As I matured, my clinical work gradually began to shift. I had been trained as a family therapist. I did brief work, 10–20 sessions with clear goals and measurable outcomes. Slowly, family referrals dwindled and adult women began to come to consult with me. Most, if not all, were survivors of horrible violence in society and in the home. I had begun, at the same time, to do research in Mexico and the United States on intimate partner violence. The women's pain, the men's guilt and sorrow, the burden of child witnesses, all began to take a toll on me. I had always been able to connect with people, but brief therapy had protected me from going too deep and staying too long.

Recovery from addiction, violence, trauma in all its forms, was a different therapeutic journey. As I joined men and women on the path to recovery, I began to dream of Corn Woman, Pacha Mama, the multiple embodiments of female deity and Spirit (Barron-Druckrey, 2008). My relationships with loved ones became more authentic. I began to find my own voice. In 2003, I said good-bye to a painful marriage, and through divorce regained the friend my first husband had once been.

I was able to bear witness to my son's anguish at the divorce, to hold his anger yet not tolerate any abuse. Over time our relationship healed. My daughter stood by me; a woman emerged from the body of a troubled adolescent. As my mother's dementia progressed and her needs grew, my brother and I became her parents. He emerged as the primary caregiver and I as the provider. In a culturally dystonic role reversal, we ensured her well-being. I let her go home to Panama after my father died so she could feel the warmth of her homeland and be surrounded by the sounds, sights, and smells she still recognized.

One night I dreamed of Corn Woman again. I was riding in a bus with my friend, colleague, and spiritual mentor. I was uncertain as to my destination, but at a particular point my friend told me it was time to get off the bus. With some trepidation I followed his advice. I began to walk on a straight and narrow paved road, bordered on both sides by resplendent yellow cornfields. The fields were endless. I felt I was being drawn to a place I had not seen before but to which I belonged. Suddenly She emerged. Tall and brown, with beautiful braids of silver and white, she smiled and beckoned me to her. I fell into her sweet embrace. Without speaking, she took my hand and led me into the field of corn. I awoke.

As my Native American healer had predicted almost a decade before, I lost my head. I did the seemingly impossible. I fell in love with a man 30 years younger. We met, loved, and married in a matter of 18 months. With him, I found home in his *panatico* (Panamanian and Costa Rican) linguistic inflections. Born in Costa Rica and having lived in Panama, he understood me in a way others could not. We were each other's cultural mirror. Guided by my Serbian-Croatian healer, I surrendered to Spirit and the power of love. I became my husband's mentor, his cheerleader, his bridge to the United States and a more balanced masculinity. His love helped me heal historical wounds and led me to feel more balanced and present.

But once again I had chosen to love a troubled man who had suffered violence in his childhood and humiliation through his multiple migrations. I could not heal him and my love was not enough. Over the brief and love-filled five years of our marriage, I realized fully who I am and what I need. If I were to have a life partner, it would need to be someone who did not need an emotional midwife. And, above all, I had to stop taking on that role, particularly if uninvited to do so.

As I sensed, and tried to cope with, the loss of my second marriage, I began to receive multiple referrals for couple's therapy. Women in pain because of the addiction of their men; Chicanas, Latinas, and European-American women who loved troubled Latino men began to call. I could sit across from them, hear their stories with compassion and respect, and draw from my courage and pain to promote balance, authenticity, mutual respect, and understanding. While I gradually accepted the end of my marriage, I worked with these couples to find ways to reconnect and to love "in the war years" (Moraga, 2000), to help them save their relationships (if they so desired) or to help them part, without destroying the friendship they once had, their children, or each other.

My clinical work became more compassionate, more present, more embodied. As I realized that divorce, and separation, and dreams unfulfilled, are other forms of migration, I could embrace my own losses and choose to live more fully in the present. My relationships with colleagues, friends, and students became more boundaried. I began to take better care of myself. I began to voice my needs.

The last dream of Corn Woman had stayed with me and carried me through the painful end of my marriage. I accepted its end. I understood my need to rescue men and sacrifice myself for love. I became aware of my own value. I no longer needed the reflection of another's gaze to see me. I am an elder, with all the attendant rights my culture prescribes. I am to be respected, revered, listened to, and protected.

Without my realizing it, my students, my son-in-law, and my extended family had begun to treat me as an elder. I became a grandmother, and at the precise moment of my first granddaughter's birth, as her head crowned while I held my daughter's hand, I felt the power of Corn Woman and the blessings of all the women in my family who came before us. I had a vision of my granddaughter Lei-Lahni as a strong runner, an athlete, a beautiful brown woman. When my second granddaughter was born 27 months later, I held my daughter's hand once again and, guided by the midwife, a Catholic nun, I welcomed Naturelle into the world with song.

I am an elder, but a modern one. I work, I travel, I teach, I dance, I love, I heal, I nurture, and I seek balance in my life. As my granddaughters grow into unique individuals who give me their love and call me *Tita,* I remember my mother's loving care toward my children and I give thanks for the blessings of being in my daughter's and her daughters' life.

On Being an Elder in My Community

While my family accords me automatically the respect my elder status affords me because I am a woman of a certain age, my professional and political community treats me with the deference my age, wisdom, and experience dictates. My clients have become more diverse—women in their 20s and early 30s who are struggling to balance work, family, career, love. They see in me a woman "who has been there" and survived. Young Latinas and other women of color (both students and clients) seek in me someone who can guide them through difficult life's stages, with complex questions of identity (gender, race, class, sexuality). They want to hear my story of migration, what helped me survive the academy, how I managed to fulfill all of the culturally expected roles (daughter, wife, mother, and now grandmother) in the war zone of social unrest, discrimination, sexism, and heterosexism. These women want not only a therapist but a mentor, a cultural broker, someone who can decode complex and changing cultural norms.

Young couples come to see me because they want the skills and experience they assume I have to help them resolve their relational conflicts. They want my help with finding love once it is lost, with learning to accept or negotiate changing cultural roles. They come to see me, as once young women sought counsel from godmothers or grandmothers, because they were elders. Older heterosexual couples come see me because they are renegotiating their relationship after the children have gone, because they are deciding whether to return "home" after 20 or 30 years living in the United States and want help in preparing for a return migration and the losses it will entail. Young Latina lesbians seek my counsel on balancing family, work, duty, and love.

I have accepted the elder role. I enjoy the conversations, the *pláticas,* with these clients and students. I listen with respect, holding their stories and feeling the emotions that are expressed while remembering the sighs and faraway looks of the elders in my family when they answered the questions posed by the young woman I once was.

I am blessed to have obtained the academic preparation and life experience that allows me to be present in the lives of others whose journey is both similar and different from mine. I have traveled and crossed geographic and cultural borders. I have learned to be me regardless of location. I have developed the ability to be attuned to other's cultures while being true to myself. I have learned that it takes a long time to reach this place of calm and peace that I know have in my life. I have learned to live in the present and enjoy the moment.

Finding Home

My parents' sacrifices afforded me an education. My own efforts to become economically independent, and the love and support of my chosen family, allow me now, in this stage of my life, the freedom to be uncoupled or to love whomever I choose.

As I reflect back on my multiple voluntary border crossings I acknowledge that with each departure and return I recaptured and integrated a piece of the soul and the self left behind during coaxed and involuntary migrations.

I am an elder, guided by the women who came before me, who suffered, who lived and died so that I could have the opportunities and freedom they did not receive. I am another link in my family's multigenerational chain, the base on which my children and their children can build their own dreams. I will continue to strive to contextualize, for my children, the genealogy of pain and resilience they too have been bequeathed. As an elder I will not hold secrets but rather share the stories and spiritual teachings I have learned along the way. These narratives can help them transform our family's history of pain into their own powerful tapestry of love and joy.

As I begin to consider retirement and the course I want my life to take, I acknowledge the choices I have, products of my education and economic privilege, yet surrender to Spirit my need to plan, to control, to be in charge. Spirit will not fail me; Corn Woman will always guide me. In the meantime, I continue to find joy in teaching, inspiration in the courage of my clients and my adult children's life choices, and hope in my granddaughters' love.

REFERENCES

Barron-Druckrey, E. (2008). *Corn woman sings: A medicine woman's dream map.* Bloomington, IN: Universe.

Falicov, C. (1998). *Family therapy with Latinos: A guide to multicultural practice.* NY: Guilford Press.

Flores, Y. (2000). My father's hands. In Alarcon, N., Lavarez, C., Behar, R., Benyamor, R., Cantu, N., Fiol-Matta, L., Flores-Ortiz, Y., & Zavella, P. (Eds.), *Telling to Live: Latina feminist testimonios* (pp. 33–38). Rodham, NC: Duke University Press.

Flores, Y. (2008). Embodying dementia: Remembrances of memory loss. In A. Chabram-Dernersesian & A. de la Torre (Eds.), *Speaking from the body: Latinas on health and culture* (pp. 31–43). Tucson, AZ: University of Arizona Press.

Hardy, K. V. (2008). Race, reality and relationships: Implications for revisioning family therapy. In M. McGoldrick & K. V. Hardy (Eds.), *Re-visioning family therapy* (2nd ed., pp. 767–84). New York: Guilford Press.

Moraga, C. (2000). *Loving in the war years.* Cambridge, MA: South End Press.

Rivera, T. (1987). *Y no se lo tragó la tierra.* (E. Vigil-Piñón, Trans.). Houston, TX: Arte Público.

The Therapist at 60, The Patient at 60: Challenges for Psychotherapy

EMILY LOEB

The Wright Institute, Berkeley, California

Women (and men) come to psychotherapy in their 50s and 60s with specific developmental issues confronting them at this stage of life. Facing the ultimate end of death is, of course, underlying all challenges at this age. There are also challenges to one's narcissistic equilibrium as each woman experiences losses and limitations. This time of life requires a reevaluation of her past and a transformation of her identity and intentions moving ahead. The author speaks of having faced these issues in her own life and her own psychotherapy, an essential process in preparation to be of use to her patients in psychotherapy. Insights are drawn from personal experience as well as from the writings of existentialist thinkers, Object Relations theorists, Jungians, and also from several poets. Two case examples illustrate these themes.

The work that we do is always hard. The work we do with women in the latter part of their lives may be especially difficult in very specific ways. A life "well-lived" often has the fulfillment of past productivity, of personal recognition, good relationships, and good memories savored. People may have vitality and physical vigor that continues into the last decades. On the other hand, the women who come to consult us for psychotherapy at this time of life may be coming with discouragement, with clinical depression, and occasionally with full-on despair.

For us older professionals in the consulting room, this work is different from that with younger people. Both the older therapist and the patient are more aware of the clock ticking away time. In reality, there is less time ahead, and some possibilities that are available for younger people are simply no longer available.

Questions arise about the deeper meanings of life: existential questions, spiritual questions. More frequently than before, there is a continuing presence of illness, of physical losses and the death of loved ones to grieve. There are often difficult relationship issues unresolved, and sometimes loneliness. In the foreground, now more than before, there are questions about what is meaningful and what is still possible. All of this requires the steady presence of the therapist/analyst, a woman who is likely wrestling with the same daunting concerns.

The potential for strong countertransference reactions is often close to the surface. How well prepared are we to face these realities, with their evocative emotions? The "healer" may strive for optimism, to promote the power of positive thinking. But what the patient needs more is to have a companion on the journey, a companion who knows this territory. The patient needs a therapist who can bear to stay present with the vulnerability, the disappointments, the losses, and the fear of the unknown.

TURNING 60: MY PERSONAL WORK

When I was nearing 60, I recognized that I was slowly withdrawing from a number of my social and professional activities. Being an extrovert by nature, it felt strange for me to choose quiet time over work and friendships. I thought I was tired, but actually I was becoming depressed. Because I always have been (and continue to be) a believer in the benefits of "the talking cure," I sought a psychoanalyst whom I trusted—intentionally a person five years older than I was—and I began an important chapter in my own later life development.

In the 40 years from age 18 on I had worked with two classically trained psychoanalysts, three family therapists, and a Reichian therapist. Not one of those therapies ever changed my basic character, but each was enormously helpful to me in those life stages. One might think that this history of a life of psychotherapy will be seized on by people who are always skeptical of psychology. This certainly happens. For me, though, each experience gave me a support system and a place to put the "unthought known" into words. Each therapeutic relationship shed new light on my sense of self, each helped me to stay conscious of my life choices and their consequences. As both a patient and a psychotherapist, I remain a strong believer in the benefits of this work. I've often told students that if they couldn't afford both graduate school tuition and personal therapy, they should undergo personal therapy first. In addition to personal therapy and good supervision, I also place great value on the authentic person of the therapist and on the accumulation of her life experience.

Over these four decades, I've learned a great deal about character structure and about conflict, defenses, and intersubjective experience. I've learned a great deal about listening for the unconscious, about transferences, about timing and interpretation. More than all the theory and practice, however, I've learned from my own life experiences. I have a deeper sense of the "human condition," more compassion, more confidence in individuals' innate resilience, and definitely a longer perspective on life's course.

AMBITIONS AND THE EGO IDEAL

When I was 60, my most immediate source of unhappiness was the disparity between my lifelong goals and the reality of my actual accomplishments. I felt successful as a psychologist, as a teacher, as a mother, but I had had other dreams, other ambitions that were now no longer possible. My self-image was shaken. Like many people, I had held an ego-ideal and unrealistic illusions about my own potential. I felt surprised, discouraged, and disappointed. Reality consisted of facts that were hard to digest. Some disappointments could be resolved only with grieving and acceptance over time.

While wrestling with all of this, I had a recurring question, which I've now heard from many in my age group: "Should I be trying to do more (as in the "use it or lose it" program)? Or should I be learning to relax, to accept doing less?" As you might predict of someone brought up in an academic/intellectual family, all this while, I tried to find answers in books. In a fashion that was typical for me, I began to read everything I could find that referred to the life passage that I was entering. I read memoirs and fiction, poetry and nonfiction, all the classics on facing aging and even facing mortality (Becker, 1975; Viorst's *Necessary Losses*, Erikson, 1959). I read psychoanalytic theorists and books by Jungians and by Buddhist teachers who were previously unfamiliar to me.

As a marvelous example of irony in action, I found the following passage in a book by the Jungian analyst Cara Barker (2000):

> "World Weary Woman" comes into the second half of life with a masculine attitude, having invested heavily in her capacity for high performance.... Goals have come from what she thinks is "reasonable," or "possible to achieve," or "should be achieved." Her intellect has structured her actions... her creativity...made servant to her ambition. She knows that she can "produce." Yet, as she ages and her need to make intimate contact with soul deepens, she notices more and more that her outer productions bring less satisfaction. [It matters less] whether the outer world rewards her efforts... [as she] struggles to come to terms with what is the center of her life. (p. 3)

When I read this, I laughed with pleasure and a shock of recognition: I was "world weary woman." As always, using my thinking function was my comfort and refuge. I knew that Cara Barker was right about the limits of intellect, but I also knew that it wasn't that simple. I had changed over the years from a person who became quickly excited with new people, with new ideas and possibilities. I was now less inclined to leap wholehearted into a new approach. Whereas my past idealizations had been so intense and all-consuming, I had also learned how often they had to be modified when realities set in causing disappointments and de-idealizations. At age 60, I actually was not so quick to accept a necessary split between intellect and "soul" (as Barker uses it). I continued to use my intellect actively and with pleasure, but I also felt more curiosity about this thing called soul. I investigated some of the teaching of Buddhist teachers. I noticed the seeming equilibrium of my friends who engage in their spiritual practices and wanted to find more of that for myself by some means.

WHERE EGO HAS BEEN, THERE SHALL BE . . . WHAT?

Questions about the place of ego were in the foreground. I thought about Freud's famous dictum "where Id is, there shall Ego be." And now my thoughts turned to the next question: "Where Ego has been, there shall . . . what? Shall be what?" In my reading, I found some provocative opinions about the place of "ego" through the stages of life development. One of the most helpful books that I read was called *The Middle Passage*, written by a writer and Jungian analyst named James Hollis (1995). His book outlines a clear developmental life course with varied challenges along the way, and his observations about the later stage of life rang loudly true to me: "Perhaps the greatest shock of all is the erosion of the illusion of ego supremacy. However successful our ego project may once have been, it can hold dominion no longer. The breakdown of the ego means that one is not really in control of (one's) life (p. 41)."

> "The Middle Passage" . . . presents us with an opportunity to reexamine our lives and to ask the sometimes frightening, always liberating, question: "Who am I apart from my history and the roles I have played?" When we discover that we have been living what constitutes a false self, that we have been enacting a provisional adulthood, driven by unrealistic expectations, then we open the possibility for the second adulthood, our true personhood . . . . [This will be] an occasion for redefining and reorienting the personality, a rite of passage between the extended adolescence of first adulthood and our inevitable appointment with old age and mortality. Those who travel the passage consciously render their lives more meaningful. Those who do not, remain prisoners of childhood, however successful they may appear in outer life. (p. 7)

Hollis continues,

> Most of the sense of crisis in midlife is occasioned by the pain of that split. The disparity between the inner sense of self and the acquired

personality becomes so great that the suffering can no longer be suppressed or compensated. What psychologists call decompensation occurs. The person continues to operate out of the old attitudes and strategies, but they are no longer effective. Symptoms of midlife distress are in fact to be welcomed, for they represent not only a grounded self underneath the acquired personality but a powerful imperative for renewal. The transit of the Middle Passage occurs in the fearsome clash between the acquired personality and the demands of the Self. A person going through such an experience will often panic and say, "I don't know who I am anymore." (p. 15)

No wonder there is such enormous anxiety. One is summoned, psychologically, to die unto the old self so that the new might be born. [This] is not an end in itself; it is a passage...to earn the vitality and wisdom of mature aging...a summons from within to move from the provisional life to adulthood, from the false self to authenticity. (Hollis, 1995, p. 15)

OLD ATTITUDES FADE: PERSONAL AND THEORETICAL CHANGES

I was very aware that Barker and Hollis were Jungians, writers who were not on my old shelf of books. Reading Hollis, I was reminded of a conversation with an old colleague many years ago. In a discussion about Freudians and Jungians, she had said to me, "Oh you know those Jungians. They never see psychopathology in people; they always imagine Healthy Striving in the most serious of emotional straits." This propensity to see healthy striving in myself and in my patients actually is true for me. That was never a point of philosophical alienation between myself and my Jungian analyst colleagues. I had always gravitated to the humanist-existential writers, but in the past I had felt an antipathy to Carl Gustav Jung and his work.

From the beginning of my education in psychology, I never had understood Jung's language or his imagery. I grew up in an extended family of Freudians and was deeply steeped in the Old Testament–like world view of Ego-Id-Superego, Oedipal conflicts with much emphasis on guilt, etc. Jung and his ideas were not well regarded in the time and place of my introduction to psychology and I had trouble understanding his alternate vocabulary of archetypes and complexes. I could never remember which was which, between "anima" and "animus." Beyond this, my personal antipathy to Jung the man and my earlier rejection of his theories had another basis. I believe that the deepest chasm has been between my own Jewish identity and Jung's behavior during the horrific years of anti-Semitism and Holocaust in Europe in the 1930s, his ideas about the Jewish race and his willing takeover of the psychoanalytic journals when the founders were barred during the Nazi era.

By the time that I was 50 and more curious to understand Jung, I also encountered the burgeoning literature (e.g., Carotenuto, 1982) that revealed his exploitative (ab)use of women throughout his life, the ones he called his muses. His use and abuse of Sabina Spielrein (early on) and his continuing relationship with Toni Wolfe caused great hurt to his loyal wife Emma for decades of their marriage. This treatment of women angered me. Jung had never learned the lessons that Freud taught when Freud observed the power differential between doctor and patient or older man and younger woman. Freud had invented the terms *transference* and *countertransference* and was attempting to build a protective structure to contain the turbulence of erotic transferences to prevent the more-powerful person (whether the analyst in a therapy or the man in a primarily male-dominated society) from abusing that power. I had had my own experiences of idealization and disillusionment with powerful men as I grew up, and in the process of seeing more than 500 women in therapy, over 37 years, I've known many women who were recovering from damaging abusive experience with men. My own experience, my feminism, and my empathy with these clients, had combined to make me so alert to and critical of Jung's love affairs with women patients and his unacknowledged use of their ideas.

As a Jew, a feminist, and a Freudian, I had a long-standing worldview that did not have much room for Carl Jung. That was true until I reached this current stage of my life. Now, unexpectedly, with all of these things remaining unchanged, my perspective seemed to open up. My earlier focus on the formative years of childhood, my Ego-Id and Superego imagery, began to dissolve. I seemed to experience some type of "meltdown" (my own experience of alchemy, perhaps) with new imagery emerging. To my surprise, I began seeing, in my 60s, that Jung and his followers were indeed on to something essential. Along with the Existentialists, they focus on the human drive to find or to make meaning and to develop the true self. This is not unlike other theorists, Winnicott or Kohut for example, but the Jungians emphasize individuation and looking forward rather than back.

The Jungian writers' understanding of the nature of introversion and extroversion, the value of "a turn within" and a need for transformations, perhaps even transcendence, has become valuable to me. Although I do not question that childhood experience forms character, I find that I'm far more interested in looking forward at this time. I work to accept what is real, to let go of nostalgia, ego, and ambition, to aim toward all that is still possible.

THE PRIMACY OF REALITY: SUFFERING, GRIEVING, ACCEPTANCE

Some familiar aspects of aging brought on my personal depression, and these same phenomena are recognized by all who write about aging. We all know that the overwhelming approach of death—now coming sooner rather than later—is the "river running through" our minds. It is possibly the stuff of frequent nakedly conscious thoughts. And we all know that waking up with painful body parts, noting an absence of sexual energy, and perhaps of energy in general, can be demoralizing and dispiriting with devastating intensity. A new day ahead looks less tantalizing than a newly dawning day looked in our youth. Many events have already occurred: many happy events, many tests passed, graduations of our own, our children's, of our students. And we probably have photos and journals of travels and adventures. It's also true that many unhappy events have occurred: significant deaths, disappointments, failures, breakups, breakdowns, wreckage of certain dreams, dissolution of illusions.

The reality we must face and metabolize is based on facts of biology, psychology, time, and space, all of the things we haven't done that will no longer be possible to do, all that we've missed and can't recover, the limitations of mind, body, resources, and time that remain, the discovery that life is not necessarily predictable or fair. New realities demand recognition, acceptance, and then rededication to the future.

During my busy year of reading, I enjoyed the wide-ranging landscape of perspectives on later life. Depending on the writer, the pendulum continually swung from the light to the dark, to the light to the dark. Among those with the darker view is Otto Kernberg. In his book *External Reality and the Internal World* (Kernberg, 1980) he wrote the following about external reality:

> The "average expectable environment" includes aggression, sadism, corruption, and envy... apart from those few who manage to live in ivory towers, we are constantly confronted with the full impact of narrow-mindedness, prejudice, envy, bias, and other forms of more or less rationalized aggression that we have to deny within ourselves. The task is to face these attacks realistically... to stand up to them without denial, masochistic submission or blind rebelliousness. (p. 128)

Kernberg is a psychoanalyst of the Object Relations School who was strongly influenced by Melanie Klein. In my own process of comparing ideas, I asked myself, "How different is this from the belief system of the Buddhists who teach that the first rule of life is Suffering?"

Fortunately, the Buddhists in their practice really do practice. They practice how to sit still and face what's real, how to refrain from running away from suffering, how to withhold judgments (of self and others), and how to practice compassion in the face of it all. Reading Hollis, I found a similar dark description of a disillusionment that has to be faced. Unlike Kernberg, Hollis locates the problem in the nature of "the universe," not in the nature of men and women among themselves. Hollis (1995) wrote:

> One of the most powerful shocks of the Middle Passage is the collapse of our tacit contract with the universe—the assumption that if we act

correctly, if we are of good heart and good intentions, things will work
out. We assume a reciprocity with the universe. If we do our part, the
Universe will comply. (p. 41)

This paragraph from Hollis resonated powerfully for me. It feels like a
concise summation of the shock and dismay that follows many tragic and
near-tragic life experiences. We all ask, Why did that happen? What could
have caused that? Where is the logic? The timeliness? The fairness? These
familiar questions have become popularized today as "why do bad things
happen to good people?" But in reality, they hark all the way back to the
Old Testament story of Job.

My own history includes the very early deaths of my younger brother,
young father, and barely middle-aged mother. For this reason, despite
growing up with a lot of material security, I never did experience the world
as safely protected by a benevolent (divine?) presence. In fact, I personally
doubted a safe "contract with the universe" from a very young age. There
are many people, however, who have not met death close up so early in life
and they usually appear to feel more surprised and more shocked when
negative events unfold.

"A GOOD OLD AGE"

"A good old age," as Helen Nearing wrote, "can be the crown of all our life's
experiences, the masterwork of a lifetime" (Nearing, 1995, p. viii). My own
tendency toward the darker view was both a useful and not-useful preparation for the dark shadows and steep steps in getting older. I did feel curious
nonetheless when I saw the book by Helen Nearing called *Light on Aging
and Dying*. The cover blurb explained that Nearing was 99 years old when
she edited this book, so it promised to offer words of wisdom from a healthy
"surviving elder."

Scott and Helen Nearing were individualists who stepped back
from various forms of social convention in their youth. They were politically
active pacifists, conservationists, crusaders, and vegetarians. After losing his
professorship, Scott and his wife Helen made their way "back to the land"
in Maine and lived the 53 years of their married life there. Together, Helen
and Scott wrote a book called *Living the Good Life*, which was inspirational
to thousands of readers.

At age 99, Helen wrote that when Scott was 100 years old, he decided
to take charge of his own death and he did so by gradually reducing his
nourishment until he died "as he chose" and "in peace." Reading this
glowing account of Scott's death, I felt envious, of course; who would not
want to live to 100 and choose the circumstances of one's own death?

I also felt unsettled, however. The Nearings's life story is so unlike that
of my own family, of my friends and of my patients in psychotherapy. It

seemed that for them the "contract with the universe" described by Hollis was indeed a reality. They lived a righteous and clean life, and they lived long and in good health. Scott and Helen Nearing were unusual in the way that they clarified their values, both political and personal, early in their lives. They lived what they believed, and they were "rewarded" with fulfillment and peace at the end of long lives. One could say that their early courage in individuation (defining themselves in difference from their predominant culture) worked out well for them. But I'm not certain what I could learn from their story at this late date. I am a woman in my 60s, and it's much too late for me to undo my years of living life in a city, eating meat, and enduring stress.

The reality of my life and the lives of my family, my friends, and my psychotherapy patients bears little resemblance to the Nearings' experience. I don't personally know anyone at all who could take control of her life or death in any way close to the Nearings. The women and men who come to see me for psychotherapy are coming with distress and confusion, chronic or acute and generated in their own process of aging.

I'll turn now to the challenge of understanding my patients, who still want to feel well and productive in these decades remaining. I could be wrong, but I very much doubt that they could find the understanding they find with me if they went to a woman who was much younger or one who had not yet walked this trail.

THE DEVELOPMENTAL TASKS OF LATER MIDDLE AGE

This accumulation of personal life experience has been invaluable for me, and I believe it's been invaluable for the women who I see, who are working through issues in their third of life. I don't see this time as a time of "deterioration" or of "winding down." I do see it as a specific developmental stage with its own specific developmental tasks. These are some of the challenges I faced, though the list is far from complete:

1. Recognition of the inevitability of death
2. Acceptance of the physical changes that come with aging
3. Development of the capacity to mourn
4. Resignation to the imperfections in one's self and others
5. Work toward reparations in relationships
6. Acceptance of dependency, independence, and interdependence
7. Acceptance of one's own life cycle as something that had to be
8. Taming of envy and cultivation of gratitude
9. Investment in new goals and pursuits, avenues of creative transformation
10. Finding sources of comfort from the external world and the "turn within" to the internal world

Frequently, in clinical case presentations, we hear about therapies with a clear beginning, a middle phase, and an ending (for public consumption, the endings are mostly Good Resolutions, with a desired outcome). I will present two examples of the kind of work that I do with women patients over 60. I want to be clear that both of these women continue to wrestle with the issues described. Neither of them, nor I myself, has arrived at a clear happy ending. I can report, nonetheless, that our work together is energetic, dynamic, and often deeply moving. At times we laugh together wryly; at times we both have tears. Sometimes we just sit together silently, feeling the pain of events that can't ever change. On other days, though, I often say, "You know, it's really not over until it's over." Surprising possibilities lie ahead, even to the deathbed of a parent, which I have seen more than once.

A CASE OF SUCCESSFUL INDIVIDUATION/PAINFUL ISOLATION

Noreen[1] came to therapy when she was 61. Tall and youthful-looking, Noreen dressed attractively and described her successful business. For over 25 years she'd done interior design and had built a loyal clientele. She'd also invested wisely, bought property, saved money, and had come close to a personal goal of having a million dollars in assets in order to finally stop working so hard and retire. Noreen described her life of hard work as comparable to one of "those horses with blinders that go round and round a circle yoked to a rope but always in motion, maybe trampling grain."

Noreen described herself as having insomnia, fatigue, and depression. She said that she wanted to "break out of the harness, to jump the fence and to run." She wanted to retire, to travel, to be free. But Noreen had realized she had no idea how to do this.

Noreen's wish to retire was far more complicated than it might have seemed at first. Early in our work we saw that a pervasive theme in Noreen's thoughts was the fear of financial failure, loss, and ruin. Although her parents had owned a successful restaurant and cocktail lounge in Baton Rouge, the business had failed eventually because of her father's alcohol addiction. It also turned out that neither her brother nor any cousins in her generation had gotten higher education nor developed a successful professional life. Noreen found it difficult to believe that she deserved her success and difficult to trust that the solid foundations built in her life would remain solid and reliable.

After months of exploring this insecurity based on internalized identifications, we arrived at the next level of difficulty standing between Noreen and retirement. This reality was her personal isolation and loneliness. Whenever she would leave work behind for holidays or vacation, Noreen was

---

[1]In the two cases I am going to present, names and identifying data have been changed.

faced with how alone she is in the world. Her living family members remained in Louisiana, and Noreen deeply missed having a family, but she could no longer identify with them or relate to them. Many cousins, nieces, and nephews were different from her in their cultural values, politics, and in their continued use of alcohol and disorganized home lives. Virtually every holiday visit back "home" ended badly with vows never to go "home" again.

I frequently shared with Noreen my view of her accomplishments as a woman virtually forced to leave home for self-preservation. She had given up home and family to build a separate identity and a viable life—essentially to save her Self. Using her fine intelligence and her ambitious drive, she escaped from the family model and broadened her world beyond theirs. In Jungian terms, she was highly successful in her ability to individuate. Less fortunately, however, Noreen continued her "self-definition" project into adult life where she was self-reliant but mostly alone. Attachments came and went very quickly as Noreen ended relationships abruptly whenever the differences between Self and Other appeared. The ability to negotiate merging and separateness, flexible boundaries, and intimacy versus isolation, completely eluded her. Over decades, she would panic and then rage in the face of relationship disappointments and then would end relationship after relationship. This pattern occurred with women friends as well as with men.

Fortunately for Noreen, this issue erupted quickly in our early work together. When I left town during a long holiday, Noreen knew how to reach me but became desperate and furious that I was unavailable when she fell into a crisis with family visiting. When we reconvened in our first New Year's appointment, Noreen "fired" me, angrily raging that I was of no use to her, that she'd been mistaken to begin attaching/depending/trusting (not her words, but her meaning). As it happened this was an ideal rupture because it made it possible for us to attend to Noreen's unmediated reaction—her all-or-nothing experience of relationship and her lifelong impulse to disconnect rapidly following disappointment—and to her lack of practice in staying in relationship to negotiate differences and disappointments.

An added layer of difficulty runs through Noreen's self-experience. Because of the anger and rage that pours out of her after disappointment and hurt, Noreen has felt for her entire life that she's basically "bad," an "ugly and mean" person. These deep-seated character issues have all been elucidated by our familiar writer-teachers in the schools of Interpersonal (Object Relations) theory, Self-Psychology, and attachment theory. Moreover, the difficult issues in Noreen's life are familiar in the lives of many of our patients.

What becomes clear in thinking about Noreen, however, is that she came to therapy at age 60, because all of her other successes still left her alone in the last chapter of her life. Freud had said that fulfillment comes through "Work" and "Love." Noreen had developed her life and self unevenly so that only the first had been possible. "Love" need not mean the accomplishment of a single intimate relationship, but it certainly refers to the possibility of trust and attachment to others. Companionship, affection, give and take, continuity of caring all had eluded Noreen, so contemplation of retirement from work brought the other void into painful relief.

By way of suggesting a plateau in Noreen's work, I will include a poem here that turned out to be deeply meaningful to her. All through our work together, Noreen had said repeatedly that her own family was so sick that she could never create a family that would seem "normal." She felt herself to be abnormal and virtually "contaminated" as she "carried" them inside her permanently. Susan Griffin's (1976) poem, however, suggested something different about the way that normal is different from ideal:

Love should grow up like a wild iris in the fields,
unexpected, after a terrible storm, opening a purple
mouth to the rain, with not a thought to the future,
ignorant of the grass and the graveyard of leaves
around, forgetting its own beginning. Love should
grow like a wild iris
but does not.

Love more often is to be found in kitchens at the dinner
hour,
tired out and hungry, lingers over tables in houses where
the walls record movements; while the cook is probably angry,
and the ingredients of the meal are budgeted, while
a child cries feed me now and her mother not quite
hysterical says over and over, wait just a bit, just a bit,
love should grow up in the fields like a wild iris
but never does
really startle anyone, was to be expected, was to be
predicted, is almost absurd, goes on from day to day, not
quite blindly, gets taken to the cleaners every fall, sings old
songs over and over, and falls on the same piece of rug
that never gets tacked down, gives up, wants to hide, is not
brave, knows too much, is not like an
iris growing wild but more like
staring into space
in the street
not quite sure
which door it was, annoyed about the sidewalk being
slippery, trying all the doors, thinking
if love wished the world to be well, it would be well.

Love should
grow up like a wild iris, but doesn't, it comes from

the midst of everything else, sees like the iris
of an eye, when the light is right,
feels in blindness and when there is nothing else is
tender, blinks, and opens
face up to the skies. (Griffin, 1976, p. 260)

Noreen is still working on the long-standing issues that interfere with
more satisfying relationships. She comes to therapy regularly, even though
many sessions are filled with dark and difficult feelings. I can say that with
my encouragement, Noreen has begun to revisit her less-than-perfect family
and has even found some pleasure in being generous with financial gifts that
she could afford and they could not. At times, Noreen, unconsciously, places
her hand on her heart when she speaks of feeling more open, being more
tolerant, feeling more connected.

ELENA'S WORK: CHALLENGES TO NARCISSISTIC EQUILIBRIUM

In striking contrast with Noreen, is Elena, who also entered therapy in her
60s. Elena grew up in Los Angeles, the eldest and favorite daughter of three,
with parents in the Hollywood film industry. Elena was praised for her looks
and her acting talent from the time she was 7 or 8 years old and was launched
by her parents on a career of performing as a child in films and live performance by age 16. Good adult judgment allowed Elena to have a virtually
normal life in her teen years.

Gifted with high intelligence, Elena enjoyed college, did well academi-
cally, and even began a doctoral program in English Literature. By the time
Elena was 25, however, she had some symptoms both of hypomanic states
and some of depression. Her memory of that period is colored by high
anxiety about having to make choices and how to make the right choice.
There was the path of academia open to her. There was the possibility of
going back into the profession of acting and directing, and there was the
opportunity to marry and settle down. Elena was courted by a man some
years older than she, who was a highly successful businessman and who
was eager to marry her.

Elena's healthy narcissism had been well fed by her adoring parents and
by her early successes. In addition, Elena has a manic disposition, tempera-
mentally, and a very high energy level, even now in her 60s. One can easily
imagine how these elements all combined so that Elena—unable to give up
any promising possibility—managed to set aside none of the choices, launch-
ing her life on a course of trying to do it all: writing, teaching, directing,
performing occasionally, marrying, raising children. It would not have been
difficult to foresee that Elena would be dramatically thrown off her course as
she reached age 60.

Menopause hit Elena very hard, physiologically and psychologically. She was a woman especially accustomed to high-riding energy and very accustomed to the pleasure of her own erotic energy, with its charge for her and its impact on others, and her sense of self was radically challenged.

The story of Elena is the story that Otto Kernberg captured with such acuity when he wrote about the challenges to narcissistic equilibrium in middle age. Kernberg (1980) includes two chapters that helped me a great deal through their clarity. The chapters are called "Normal Narcissism in Middle Age" and "Pathological Narcissism in Middle Age." I had been wrestling with these issues in my own psychoanalytic therapy, and this work served me well when I saw Elena as a patient.

Kernberg's language is fairly technical, using the vocabulary of Object Relations theory and building on Kleinian ideas about envy and gratitude. The following quote is from the chapter on pathological narcissism in which he describes the difficulties of patients who cling to past successes, illusions, grandiosity, and feelings of omnipotence. He describes the problems of patients who rebel against the realities of age and change and can't move toward realism, grieving and acceptance.

> What is received from the outside, particularly admiration, reconfirms the narcissistic gratification of the grandiose self. Admiration is "extracted" with an unconscious greed that empties the source of pleasure and gratification, which, once emptied, is left valueless. This extraction also fuels the tendency to depreciate and devalue others, particularly those who have been emptied, who now seem mediocre, inferior, or useless.... The devaluation protects the patient against envy, but at the price of a pervasive subjective sense of emptiness.... Success, applause, and admiration, once received, are absorbed and yet, strangely enough, soon become "spoiled."...[The patient] longs for a new narcissistic "refueling," but discovers that lasting satisfaction is never to be found.... Paradoxically, past success or satisfactions are a double threat: insofar as they raised expectations, they create the potential threat that the future will not live up to the past and that narcissistic aspirations, therefore, will be shattered ... at bottom, the narcissistic middle-aged patient is painfully envious of [himself or herself] in the past, having had what [he or she] no longer has.
>
> Unconscious aggression and rage...frustrations...and envy...fill the emotional life of this person as [he or she] faces the normal, predictable limitations and losses that come with getting older. (Kernberg, 1980, p. 136)

In Elena's life in her 60s, there was no diminution of the love that her husband, her children, her friends and her colleagues expressed to her. Elena suffered, nonetheless, in a torment of fury and bleakness with regard to her own self-identified "failures," with an exaggerated sense of bitterness and alienation from others, who had little ability to dislodge her from the self-torturing cycle.

It would be impossible to summarize the years and the stages of psychotherapy with Elena. Suffice it to say that our work has been long and intense. Not different from much of our work with many patients: making the unconscious conscious, encouraging affective expression, giving names to what exists and is real. In the work with Elena, the major difficulty was always within the transference relationship in which she felt, with me, competitive, envious, alternately idealizing and devaluing. In this work, I was much aided by my own earlier journey through similar turbulent waters. It was also eased at times by a shared sense of humor, including a shared sense of the insanities and inanities of our shared world.

To leave this story of Elena's work in her 60s, I'll describe a recent "plateau" on her path. With some surprise to herself, Elena found it possible to withdraw from her usual extroverted social life for several months. During these months, Elena was able to tolerate time that she spent alone with herself. She was able to complete a one-act play during this time and she was acceptably (for her) satisfied with this work. Subsequently, the play was produced at a small local theater by an amateur cast. Although Elena continued to devalue her "mini-work," as she insisted on calling it (and the amateur cast who performed it), she tolerated this creative work. The work was smaller and quieter in every way than that of her past more grandiose fantasies. In this creative work, however, Elena did overcome a period of hopelessness and "stagnation" (as Erikson would call it) and she did come alive in her modest (and quite lovely) piece of work.

CONCLUSION

As for me, still reading, thinking, sorting, working at 68, I've learned a great deal. I feel calmer, happier, still busy and involved. Between quiet times and active times, some balance is developing. I still read fiction, nonfiction, psychoanalysts, and Jungians and Buddhists, but often the most comforting reading for me is with the poets. So many condense so much in few words and one feels "met" so often with them.

Frank Bidart (2007) has a collection of poems called *Star Dust*. Near the end of "The Third Hour of the Night," a voice speaks:

> After sex & metaphysics . . . what?
> What you have made.
> Many creatures must
> Make, but only one must seek
> Within itself what to make. (p. 38)

And from another piece by Bidart (2007), titled "Advice to the Players":

There is something missing in our definition, vision, of a human being: the need to make.
We are creatures who need to make.
Because existence is willy-nilly thrust into our hands, our fate is to make something—if nothing else, the shape cut by the arc of our lives.
Making is the mirror in which we see ourselves.
But being is making: not only large things, a family, a book, a business, but the shape we give this afternoon, a conversation between two friends, a meal... (p. 10)

REFERENCES

Barker, C. (2000). *World weary woman*. Toronto: Toronto Universities Press.

Becker, E. (1975). *The denial of death*. New York: The Free Press.

Bidart, F. (2007). *Star dust*. New York: Farrar, Straus & Giroux.

Carotenuo, A. (1982). *The secret symmetry*. New York: Random House.

Erikson, E. (1959). *Identity and the life cycle*. New York: International Universities Press.

Griffin, S. (1976). *Like the iris of an eye*. New York: Harper & Row.

Hollis, J. (1995). *The middle passage*. Toronto, Canada: University of Toronto Press.

Kernberg, O. (1980). *Internal world and external reality: Object relations applied*. Northvale, New Jersey: Jason Aronson.

Nearing, H. (1995). *Light on aging and dying*. Gardiner, ME: Tilbury House Publishers.

Viorst, J. (1986). *Necessary losses*. New York: Simon and Schuster.

Aging With My Clients

SARALIE PENNINGTON

*Private Practice in San Francisco and School of Social Work at
San Francisco State University, California*

*As the therapist and client age together during the course of
psychotherapy, an array of new opportunities arise for deep
psychological work. Long-term relational, intersubjective, and
feminist therapy throughout the adult life cycle facilitates and
encourages exploration of the scope and intensity of human
experience: attachments and fear of abandonment, grief and loss,
illness and disability, spiritual connection or its absence, and the
aging process itself in all its dimensions. The author explores with
six of her clients their impressions of self, of the therapist, and of the
therapy relationship. Case material illustrates their experiences
with one another as therapist and client in therapies that have
continued from 18 to 28 years. The mutual trust and the clients'
feelings of safety and containment in the context of the therapy
relationship are reflected in their words. The author expresses deep
gratitude for this precious trust.*

I have been a social worker/psychotherapist for over 40 years, and I have
been consciously integrating my feminist self into my psychotherapy,
community organizing, and teaching since 1971, when I became part of
one of the first feminist therapy collectives in the country here in San
Francisco, where I have lived and worked for 38 years.

My feminist therapy/therapy and spiritual/political connections and
activism broadened in scope throughout these years. Approximately six
years ago, the peer consultation group of which I was a part began to explore

aging as it intersected with our psychotherapy practices. We have been fortunate to be able to present our papers at both national conferences and in local venues through the years. We recognize that our work reflects not only our professional experience but is also defined by where we are, as individuals, in the life cycle.

Writing this paper has further opened the opportunity for me to focus on something of keen interest: my own aging, and women aging, as part of the fabric of psychotherapy and feminism. As women therapists become elders, we assert that our value to the community increases. After years of working in our own therapies, consultations, and clinical relationships, each of us has traveled a unique, complex, personal and professional life journey. We know more about healing than ever before, and more about suffering as well, and we are exploring how our conceptualizations of healing, suffering, and loss can change as we age.

As the population ages in the 21st century, we will also age with our clients. By the year 2020, people 60 years and older will comprise a little less than 20% of the national population. Some of us have witnessed or have been leaders in the transition of our field from a male defined and dominated one to one with a feminist consciousness, and then into what some call a feminized profession. As women therapists, we will be presented with the opportunity to make explicit, affirm, question, and perhaps redefine the aging process with ourselves and our clients. We may modify how we conceive of therapy itself as we age in American society.

Central to these therapeutic tasks is our exploration of the transference, countertransference, and the intersubjectivity of our collective internalized ageism and sexism. We are doing this in what seems an increasingly antifeminist political climate. The process of sharing our ideas can be energizing and exciting. This work is affirming, and it validates the strength and joy of older women's invaluable creativity and wisdom. It is work that has the power to influence and change our world.

OUR CLIENTS' VIEW OF LONG-TERM THERAPY AND AGING

I have had, and continue to have, the privilege of working in therapy with many clients for many years. I have maintained a therapy relationship with several women for more than 20 years, and will share our collective experiences—including those of clients who are younger than myself, those of clients roughly my own age who have aged right along with me, and those of significantly older women who feel they are at the end stages of their life's journey.

My intent is to focus on aging with a particular emphasis on attachment, loss, and change, by looking at my client's experience, my experience, and our collective experiences in the therapy hour. However,

I wanted this to be a feminist process and did not want to assume that I knew what my clients would be feeling and thinking about these issues without first consulting them. I approached six clients with whom I have worked from 18 to 28 years and who range in age from 48 to 85 to explore our ideas. I approached only those clients who I knew would be comfortable with this process. I also did not want this interest of mine to compromise their therapy in any way, so I arranged meetings with them that were separate from their therapy. Each client who I approached was very interested in participating. Two clients were concerned that their identities would be protected. My approach was to use a loose format of open-ended questions about issues of aging. I was interested in how they feel about themselves as they age, whether our therapy has had an impact on their aging, and whether my clients have any feelings about me and my aging process. I will attempt to present a composite of responses and reactions, highlighting some individual or unique concerns.

Reconceptualizing Therapy

All of these clients, as they are growing older, have been revising the way they conceptualize therapy. They've done this in a parallel process with me, but until this undertaking no one had acknowledged it. The cornerstone of this revision is that their therapy and their relationship with me is not viewed as finite; they view it and me as a part of their lives and therapy as a part of who they are.

All of these women feel that I am as permanent and necessary as family and experience profound attachment to me. I, myself, have eased into a comfortable acceptance of the necessary place that long-term therapy, without end, can have in our lives, as therapists in our own therapy and with our clients. Looking to a therapist for cures and trying to provide them is no longer the issue. To quote one client:

> Having a therapist for many years gives me a comfort level, a deep connection that gives me the security of knowing that I am known deeply, that my conflicts and crises are immediately recognized and understood and accepted. The process is part of my life and I want it there. It is not about change but it is about me and how I see myself. You are my ally, a resource . . . you know me, see me and understand.

For others, therapy has been, at different times in their lives, a source of their survival: "Part of why I feel so vulnerable is that it is a new feeling for me to know you are not leaving me. I do not have anyone else in my life with whom I have such trust . . . this is the deep work we are doing."

An issue for everyone is the concern that we are all getting older and that I could die before they do, which creates varying levels of anxiety.

The level of anxiety seemed to be related to the level of meaningful connection in their lives. "It's a real love, so I dread the loss of it . . . . Who will I go to, to cope with the loss of you? It's like losing my compass."

What seems clear to me is that our clients are not abandoning or finishing therapy as they age. As long as we are able and continue to work, we will have the opportunity to accompany our clients on their journeys. All feel supported by my age and experience and feel they relied on it when experiencing the difficult deaths of parents, siblings, spouses/partners, friends, and relationships. Those who were aware of my own losses, particularly the sudden loss of my mother, felt strengthened by my experience, especially those who were concerned that I might not be present for them while sustaining these losses.

The Impact of Therapy on Clients' Aging

Five of the six clients viewed their lives as emerging and unfolding during the course of our therapy. All feel they have become/are becoming more authentic and more aware and conscious of how they affect others. They feel that they have many choices, both internal and external, that come from a deep understanding of self. Some feel that they have come into adulthood in the course of therapy. For one client my feminism and complete acceptance of her being gay has been essential for our work together.

Another client felt that the downside or discouraging aspect of therapy for her is that certain issues have not gotten better over time, and she spends a fair amount of time being angry with me: "You said that my terror would get less intense, and why hasn't this happened?" She said that she needed to trust me over time and allow me to hold the hope for her, in the face of this terror. Since the initial writing of this material, this client's terror has diminished, both in frequency and duration.

Still another confided:

> I am offended by my dependency. If you were not my best friend, I'd
> have blown you off. . . . I feel subtly coerced to continue because of
> the boundaries that protect the relationship, as I know you would not
> continue to see me if I stopped therapy. Yet our relationship would
> not have developed without boundaries, if I had not been sure enough
> of your limits. I have my own boundaries and my need for them too.

This client is now 76 and we have worked together for 18 years. A woman who has lived a seriously traumatic life complete with diagnoses of major depression and borderline personality disorder, she has, in just the past few months, made a momentous internal shift. "I don't want you to think you can take the credit but I finally realize that I can depend on our relationship and don't need to constantly force myself on other people, then become furious when they set limits and then I screw the whole thing up." Telling me that I would be proud of her, she also stated that she reached out to a former dear friend she completely "blew off" five years ago after a disagreement. Up until this moment she had taken pride in never reaching out like this, being very clear that the other would always have to come to her after such a disruption. I am truly moved by this client who, after burning most all of her relational bridges, is now able to truly and genuinely open herself to new possibilities.

All view me as a role model, even the clients who are older than me, and feel very connected when discussing menopause, health issues, critical illness, death and dying, and aging parents, spouses, partners, and other relatives. For some, I have been able to suggest resources that I knew, or perhaps even used, and this has added to the feeling of protection, connection, and safety.

All feel they are aging more positively due to the development of our relationship and their growth in therapy. All feel the desire to redefine aging for themselves and others. They see many options. They do not feel predestined to age like their parents (none experienced their parents as aging well) and see richness even from the experience of pain and loss. I, of course, have been enriched and strengthened spiritually and intellectually from the incredible experiences in therapy with these women.

Several clients are aware that it can be difficult to find older wisdom, and some want to be part of a process of creating that wisdom. If feminism has not shaped them, it has had an influence on their lives. All are annoyed or angry about how women are increasingly devalued as we age and see ageism and sexism joining forces with which we must not collude. They feel ongoing support and encouragement to be open to change and creativity in all aspects of their lives and to desire intimacy and/or intensity in their relationships.

Aging-Related Physical Changes in the Therapist and Client

I was curious about the impact on therapy of my physical process of aging, about how I appeared to my clients. This discussion put me and my clients in a particularly vulnerable situation. Did they notice that I had grown older over the years that we had been together? To me, some of my clients seem frozen in time, in appearance and even age, until I come to grips with the years. All of these women have talked about their physical changes and changing appearance with me, including clients going through mastectomy, radiation and chemotherapy, loss of vision, and debilitating musculoskeletal problems.

Physical change is generally presented to me by my clients as something to be dreaded, conquered, or having to accept. Occasionally during a session, a client may have commented generally favorably on how I look. However, one client actually has told me more than once how much better I would look if I had just a little facelift, that it would take years off my life.

When I explicitly raised the issue of my own physical changes with these clients, the responses varied. There was actually not much notice, or concern, or interest in my physical aging. One client said she thought I was a little more forgetful about times and dates, but then again it might be her own faulty memory because she too was aging, and that yes she noticed my face had changed but that she liked how it was changing. Another said that there were few observable changes, that she noticed a difference about 10 years ago when I went from being lineless to having lines. "You have the same warm and radiant eyes when I walked into your office eighteen years ago and said 'this is my therapist'... an instant role model." She added that she wishes she could be like me when she's 65: "You are absolutely gorgeous." Another had a picture of me from perhaps 15 years ago, and when she looked at it she realized that my face had changed, had obviously gotten older, but otherwise she did not think about it. When she does, she likes to think of me as a wise and loving grandmother, which brings her comfort.

So I hypothesize that the longer we work together, the less important the exterior, the less noticed and necessary it is as a marker. Both client and therapist, having regular ongoing contact, do not seem to change. The external change they do see tends to be given a positive interpretation.

THE PRIVILEGE OF AGING TOGETHER

If our clients tend to "see" our aging as positive, we then have the opportunity to be part of a collective positive redefinition of aging. For each client, the meaning of my aging and my physical changes, or what they notice and what is important to them, is different. For one, it is perhaps frightening; she sees me mirroring her changes and fears the ultimate loss. For others my changes are inspiring or comforting.

It has been, and continues to be, a privilege to do long-term therapy and to be aging with my clients. I would like to share a quote from a holiday message from my eldest client, who is in her 80s, and who has recently been diagnosed with dementia. It confirms and validates how psychotherapy—over time, as we age and as our clients age—continues to not only heal but also to be part of an ongoing process of growth and creativity:

> This year is almost over and so much has happened.... I really and truly don't know how I would have made it through without the many years of your help, understanding, and guidance... giving me the support and strength to follow through. It's been a long struggle and an awakening for me.... I am with hopes that I will stay well, and keep my spirits

up, and continue on my journey, and go back to enjoying many of my cultural activities, and seeing friends, and doing what I can to help others too. I hope the New Year will be a new beginning for me.

I realize that I am "coming out" to you rather fearlessly as a very long-term therapist, which in some circles would be highly controversial. I also realize that what I've explored and written sounds so positive and so productive. Perhaps what I am communicating is the deep satisfaction that comes from the strength and beauty of the relationship that we develop in this long-term work that allows us the remarkable privilege to not only go on our client's life journeys but to also be an influential part of those journeys.

To ensure that this work will continue, feminist therapists will need to focus our political efforts to ensure that Medicare and other benefits will continue to be resources that can meet the needs of our clients, and we will need to be involved in establishing affordable feminist-oriented therapy opportunities for older women so that we can continue to heal, grow, and create all the days of our lives.

Finding My Professional Voice: A Woman of Color's Professional Journey

HARRIET CURTIS-BOLES

*California School of Professional Psychology at Alliant International University,
San Francisco, California*

Through a process of self-reflection this article traces my professional development starting with my early training and professional socialization and ending with my current treatment philosophy and clinical practice in my work with women. I empha-size the impact of my gendered upbringing and social position as a woman of color as I chronicle the struggles, and ultimate solutions, to finding my professional voice in White, male-dominated institu-tions. These struggles included reconciling my cultural knowledge and lived experience with my formal training, and included estab-lishing legitimacy and credibility in my perspectives and expertise. The wisdom of my later years allowed me to liberate myself from the "voices" of theorists, instructors, and supervisors from the past, to become my own authority and to integrate my spiritual values and important lessons learned from being a mother into my work with clients. The process of this transformation is described.

In our youth-oriented culture, aging is often characterized as something to be dreaded and is associated with decay and decline (Cavanaugh & Blanchard-Fields, 2002; Vaillant, 2008). Women are encouraged to "mask" their aging through the application of topical creams, toxic injections, or cosmetic surgery. How often have you heard the phrase, "Never ask a woman her age"? We have been taught to fear and despise the aging process, forever mourning the losses of our youth.

Some adult developmental theories redefine the later stages of life to include opportunities for positive change and growth, in self-representation as well as in one's relationships to others and the world (Colarusso & Nemiroff, 1981; Settlage, Curtis, Lozoff, Silberschatz, & Simburgm, 1986). Erik Erikson (1950) emphasized the capacity for generativity and integrity (versus stagnation and despair) in the middle and later adult years, while Levinson (1978) focused on achievement, creativity, and retrospective self-reflection. Recognizing that these early adult development theories were based primarily on the experiences of men, other theorists identified the distinctive characteristics of women's development, anchoring our socialization in relationship-building and maintenance, caregiving, and personal sacrifice (Gilligan, 1982; Josselson, 1978; Lippert, 1997).

As I think back over my professional journey, I am aware that my course was significantly influenced by my gendered upbringing and my social positions as a woman and as a person of color. The path of my professional socialization is not unlike that of many women who have written about this experience, who have struggled to find their voice in a White, male-dominated culture and to reconcile the demands of their professional lives with their personal values. In a study on women leaders, Lustgarten (2008) wrote about women's experience of internal and external obstacles to realizing and manifesting their personal power and capacities, including fears of speaking up and not being included, lack of self-trust, and the absence of cultural and societal validation. These women typically found their "voice," owning and articulating their personal wisdom, in the second half of life, in the years between 40 and 60.

The narratives of women of color who have addressed professional socialization and development in academic and work settings reveal common themes of invisibility, alienation, and devaluation (Alfred, 2001; Black & Magnuson, 2005; Bryant et al., 2005; Souto-Manning & Ray, 2007). Successful women of color, interviewed in their 40s through their 80s (Alfred, 2001; Black & Magnuson, 2005), reported that establishing legitimacy and credibility in their careers was a process that "developed over time" and involved fighting against concerns about their competency, feeling and being treated like an outsider, and not having their perspectives valued.

As I think back over my own professional development, many of the struggles these women expressed resonate with my own experience. Consistent with theories of adult development, and mirroring the stories of women's professional journeys, my later years have fostered and nurtured a sense of wisdom, confidence, and liberation that have made my personal and professional connections deeper, richer, and more meaningful.

I will present to you a collection of self-reflections that will take the reader through the process of my professional development as an African-American woman. Though the primary objective is to share knowledge, insights, and transformations that have occurred in my latter years, given my psychodynamic training and orientation, I believe no one can be fully understood without an appreciation of their history. I have separated my personal journey toward finding my professional voice into three phases: my early training and professional socialization, a transitional period of self-recovery, and personal validation and developments in later life (my mid-40s to early 50s) that allowed for the integration of the personal and professional in my clinical work. I will end by discussing how my development has informed my clinical practice and provide recommendations for how women of color can be supported in their development as clinicians.

EARLY TRAINING AND PROFESSIONAL SOCIALIZATION

I did my doctoral training at a predominantly White university in the western part of the United States. My graduate career as a student in the late 1970s and early 1980s predated the multicultural movement in clinical psychology, though the institution I attended was considered exemplary in their commitment to diversity. The core faculty in the Clinical Psychology Department included an African-American man and a White woman, and the six students in my entering class included three ethnic minority women. This diversity in representation was set in the context of a traditional curriculum anchored in a psychoanalytic perspective. Though there were recognized experts in minority psychology on the faculty, the presentation of varying worldviews, cultural values, and practices was limited.

Lessons in the Dominant Worldview

As a student, I struggled with reconciling my personal experience and reality with what was being taught in the classroom. Having been raised in a single-parent family with a strong religious tradition, I inwardly cringed when families headed by strong Black women were categorically labeled as dysfunctional, the closeness of families like mine were characterized as enmeshed, and faith-based practices were considered a defensive rather than adaptive response to life problems.

Scheurich (1993) suggested that the best way for minority groups to receive recognition, acceptance, and rewards is to learn and reproduce the ways of the dominant group. As a young developing professional, eager to please and excel, I attempted to integrate and internalize what I was being taught as my own. Though many of the theories and principles I learned did not resonate with my experience, I voiced no objections, mastered the language, and applied accepted concepts in my academic and clinical work. In the course of my graduate work I experienced an ongoing tension between my personal cultural knowledge, based on my lived experience and "home training," and the largely monocultural, Eurocentric perspective of my academic institution.

Refuge and Restoration

I found myself growing distant from my cultural roots and sought a place where my identity as an African-American woman and developing professional could be affirmed. In discussing the challenges of African-American women in White academic and occupational institutions, Alfred (2001) referred to these places of refuge and restoration as a safe space. I found my safe space in a small community mental health outpatient center run by an African-American woman and serving the local African-American community. Here I learned the skills to work clinically with African-American clients in a context that appreciated and understood the cultural complexities of this community and how racism and classism could interface with a client's clinical presentation.

This provided some balance in my clinical training and a place where my personal, culturally informed impressions and intuitions were validated and expanded, but I kept it separate from my experience at the university. Though personally valuable, I never felt what I was learning in this community-based setting would be accepted or affirmed in my academic institution.

My outpatient internship experience at a well-respected psychoanalytic treatment center mirrored the limitations of my earlier clinical training. Though strong on traditional theory and skills development, the setting lacked a cultural perspective and orientation. I remember sitting in countless case conferences where clients of color were described as guarded and withdrawn and culturally specific experiences and behavior were pathologized. The trainers and supervisors, who were predominantly male and White, failed to consider clients' presentations in a cultural context and seemed to have never heard of Grier and Cobbs' (1968) concept of "healthy cultural paranoia" or to appreciate the dynamics of cultural transference and countertransference (Ridley, 2004). In defense of both my clinical education and training, I want to reiterate that multiculturalism had not yet appeared as a significant influence in the theory and practice of professional psychology, and the shortcomings identified here were typical of mainstream institutions at this time.

TRANSITION: SELF-RECOVERY AND PERSONAL VALIDATION

Bell hooks (1989), a Black feminist scholar, talked about self-recovery as vital to the sanity, survival, and liberation of African-American women. She asserted that to restore wholeness and integrity to our personal and professional lives, we must honor our history, give legitimacy to our wisdom and knowledge, and assume authority in representing our realities. We must find our own voices and live and speak our own truth.

Establishing My Own Sense of Confidence

My path of self-recovery followed a course of first establishing my own sense of confidence in my knowledge and expertise, which allowed a later integration of all the aspects of my multiple social identities into my professional life so that when I entered the therapy room I was relating to my clients as a "whole" person.

As a professional lacking the benefit of a mentor, I had to forge my own career path. In addition to my work as the clinical director of a mental health outpatient agency, I found a comfortable niche in a private practice serving predominantly African-American women. At my agency setting, I had the authority to hire a diverse staff and to develop a clinical training program that I felt was inclusive and respectful of cultural difference. Though I was confident in my expertise working with African-American clients, I was limited in my knowledge of other cultural minority groups since my education and training had not provided this foundation. In addition, my reach as a clinician was largely limited to my agency and private practice, where my expertise was neither tested nor challenged.

Experiencing Validation from the Profession

Though a few actions by the profession of psychology had espoused the importance of cultural diversity in clinical training and treatment (e.g., the American Psychological Association's Vail Conference of 1973 and the APA Division 17 proposal of cross-cultural competencies in 1982), it could be argued that the multicultural movement's first significant foray into professional psychology was in 1986. It was at this time that the American Psychological Association's (APA) Accreditation Committee for doctoral programs in psychology first required that training address the development of competence in conducting therapy with diverse populations. APA followed this crucial step in 1992 by the establishment of Domain D, which articulated specific diversity standards in education and practice and gave an explicit directive that compliance to these standards be documented when graduate programs applied to APA for accreditation. In 1999, Pedersen identified multiculturalism as the "Fourth Force" in psychology, emphasizing the central role of culture across and within existing theories.

The multicultural movement was particularly significant for me, personally, in several ways. Ii questioned the universality of traditional theories and practices. It advocated for an approach in education, training, and practice that incorporated multiple worldviews and cultural realities. It provided opportunities for expanding my cultural knowledge. For the first time in my professional career, I'd found a paradigm that resonated with my views on human development, mental health and illness, and clinical practice.

This validation empowered me to become more public and vocal in my perspectives on culture and clinical treatment, which eventually led to my training others about culturally competent practice.

DEVELOPMENTS IN LATER LIFE: INTEGRATION OF THE PERSONAL AND PROFESSIONAL

Two very important events happened in my late 40s to early 50s that dramatically changed my clinical practice. The first involved becoming comfortable with my spirituality in the clinical arena. The second involved finding myself with an "empty nest," with my only child completing college and establishing her home in a city hundreds of miles away.

My Spirituality

Though I have always been a very spiritual person, for many years I struggled with how to integrate spirituality into my clinical practice. I was "raised in the church," and prayer is a daily source of comfort and coping in my life. Many years ago, I had begun the practice of praying silently for my clients in particular distress. At the same time, I remained hesitant to bring spirituality directly into my clinical work. This hesitation was in direct contrast to personal transformations I have experienced, which have required a combination of psychological insight, spiritual connectedness, and behavior change. All of these elements together have been essential for positive growth in my life.

My multicultural training cautioned me not to impose my values on others, and my traditional clinical training frowned on the integration of spirituality and clinical practice. I carry the visible evidence of my race and gender into the therapy room but had the choice whether to reveal my religious identity.

I have always worn a cross, and had felt conflicted about whether to keep it visible when I work with clients. Showing this religious symbol was initially a conflict for me, out of concern for what it might elicit in my clients, what assumptions and values they might attribute to me because of my religious background that could impact the treatment. Would clients view me as conservative and intolerant and leave important material out of our work—for example, discussions of substance use and sexual activity—for fear of being judged?

I realized, on reflection, that even at this point in my career, I continued to be strongly influenced by the "voices" of theorists, instructors, and supervisors from my past. The power of these old "voices" made acknowledging and talking about spirituality in therapy taboo. On the other hand, I was aware that my spirituality is a core aspect of my identity that contributes to my strengths as a therapist: my humility, compassion, looking for and connecting to the good in others, and treating others with respect and love.

A few years ago I started wearing my cross openly and have noticed no differences in how, or the extent to which, clients address sensitive topics. This reinforced what I had learned in my training and had experienced in practice: that clients' abilities to discuss difficult issues are facilitated by the therapist's willingness to ask and support them in this process. What did change with my change was the frequency with which my clients brought their spiritual practices and beliefs into treatment and my comfort in asking about and exploring these issues. I witnessed what Kenneth Pargament (2007) asserted: "clients would welcome us into their spiritual home if we knocked on the door" (p. 16).

It was not until I felt confident in my skills as a therapist that I was able to reflect on and resolve my conflict about spirituality and practice. It is important to note though, that confidence was only one layer of this complex transformation. Other internal shifts occurred simultaneously. I had become more thoughtful about my practice, noticing not only *what* I was doing but also *why* I was doing it. I began to question who, and what, I was holding myself and my work accountable to. I realized the "inner critic" and standard-bearer for my performance was my traditional clinical training, which had shaped my expertise but also limited me in important ways. In turning inward and attending to the wisdom of my "head *and* heart" (Lustgarten, 2008) I was able to let go of the fear of judgment in showing my "true self" to clients. I emerged from this process of self-assessment and reflection with greater trust in my intuition and greater reliance on my "inner voice" to guide my clinical work. This has allowed me to be more authentic and fully engaged.

The Empty Nest

I had my first child at the age of 31, which was considered "late" by the standards of my culture and family. During my daughter's childhood years my professional life and professional development took backstage to my role as mother. Though I was invested in doing good work, much of my emotional time and energy were invested in my growing child— the falls on the playground, her first heartbreak, and the many joys of watching her develop and mature. When she entered her late teens and became more independent, shifting more of my focus to my work was a natural progression of our individuation process. Although I was still actively engaged in parenting, this marked the beginning of many lessons in "letting go" that ultimately had a significant impact on my clinical practice.

As I watched my daughter grow up and grow away, I learned many things. I realized that I could not protect her from pain and suffering. But more importantly, allowing her to struggle and find her own way made her a stronger and more capable individual. I learned to let go of my vision of who I wanted her to be and to embrace who she was choosing to become. This meant accepting differences in values and also releasing my investment in specific outcomes—whether this was about career, relationships, or where she chose to live. I reevaluated my perspective on what was important with regard to "my legacy" as a parent, what my daughter would internalize or take away from our relationship. She taught me to appreciate that being loved, valued, respected, and given the freedom of choice without the burden of judgment were my most important gifts to her.

These lessons were reflected in my clinical work as I recognized, with greater clarity, the strength and resilience of my clients. I was newly aware of the importance of supporting them in finding their own answers, keeping my assumptions and aspirations for them in check. I moved from my maternal pull to "fix" and rescue and instead entered into the clinical relationship as a true collaborator.

MY CLINICAL WORK

The unique perspective afforded to me as a woman of color, combined with the insights I have gained through introspection and liberating myself from the strictures of my traditional training, have resulted in a treatment approach emphasizing personal empowerment and self-efficacy.

My current clinical practice is at a women's college counseling center, where I work with women of varying ages and ethnicities, heterosexuals and sexual minorities, as well as women from diverse social class backgrounds. As a woman of color, I know personally the pain of race and gender discrimination and of being in a position of marginalization. As a woman, I was well socialized into the role of caregiver. I am accustomed to and find it easy to attend to the needs of others: to lend my intellect in problem solving and to lend my heart in the face of emotional pain. In contrast to my earlier associations of caregiving with protecting and taking charge, my growth as a mother helped me to realize that lasting change is facilitated by support, validation, and trust in an individual's ability to face and overcome obstacles.

Additional insights of my later years, reached through self-reflection and personal assessment, helped me to trust my instincts and be guided by my personal wisdom. The integration of these personal life experiences with my professional skills shapes my clinical practice. As an agent of change, I work to help clients find the answers within and to heal themselves. Key components of my work include helping clients find their personal voice, breaking the barriers of emotional oppression, and using a strength-based orientation.

Finding "Voice" and Breaking the Barriers of Emotional Oppression

Over the years that I have worked with women I've seen a number of commonalities and patterns in their clinical presentation. Often these clients enter treatment with voices that have been silenced and/or distorted by histories of psychological and physical abuse in important relationships. These relationships include those with parents from childhood as well as intimate relationships in their adult lives. As a result of these damaging relationships, many do not trust the validity of their own experience and come into treatment with years of yielding the scripting of their personal stories to those who have dominated and oppressed them. They tend to internalize the source of their problems (i.e., what's wrong with *me?*) even when they are intellectually aware that harmful relationships from the past have shaped their difficulties in the present. Though ambivalent, they tend to be dependent on others to tell them what to do and look outside themselves for verification of their self-worth, answers, and solutions to their problems, ultimately giving up their personal agency and control of their lives.

My work to empower women with these dynamics translates into a number of specific strategies. First I attempt to give them back their voices by helping them to reclaim and rescript their personal stories. I focus them on their inner experience of events in their lives and support their feelings as valid. I believe that if they feel empowered to speak their truth with me, this may transfer to relationships in the outside world.

I strive to provide a corrective emotional experience by creating a relationship in the therapy room that is different from what they experienced with important others in the past. To this end I attempt to be authentic and genuine in my interactions, which may include occasionally crying with a client, giving a supportive hug, and the judicious use of self-disclosure, actions that were considered taboo in my traditional training.

Strength-Based Orientation

I assume a strength-based (versus pathologizing) stance, both in my interactions with clients as well as in my clinical conceptualizations. I resist diagnostic labeling and strive to place the person before their clinical condition by thinking of my clients as women who are challenged by their circumstances as opposed to women who are weak or inadequate. I look for opportunities to reframe clients' struggles into triumphs by emphasizing their resilience, their real-life accomplishments, and their ability to cope. This does not mean minimizing or trivializing their pain or the seriousness of their circumstances, but it does mean helping them to see their situation with a different lens, attempting to replace despair with hope, and their self-defeating patterns with healthy ones. I hold for them the belief in their capacity to confront and overcome their problems and a sense of optimism about their future, until they are able to internalize these themselves.

A Case Example

A case example can illustrate my clinical approach. Mary is a 42-year-old African-American woman who started graduate school after having two children. She has a son who is 8 and a daughter 12 years of age. Mary entered treatment to address the stress of balancing school and family life. Significant events from her history include her abandonment by a drug-addicted father at the age of 5 and the limited availability of her mother, who struggled with a debilitating physical illness throughout her childhood. Due to her mother's illness, Mary was raised primarily by her maternal grandmother. Though she described her grandmother as a loving and devoted parent, she reported growing up feeling "something was wrong with her" and that she was "toxic" to people she loved.

In treatment, Mary was plagued by self-doubt, questioning if she "was good enough" for graduate school and feeling that she was being selfish and was sacrificing her family's well-being by choosing to return to school. She had a pattern, in relationships, of self-denial and frustration. She held herself to unyielding and perfectionistic standards in both her academic and personal lives. Mary was living a script shaped by failed relationships with her parents for which she assumed inordinate responsibility, leaving her feeling deficient and inadequate.

I worked to adjust Mary's unrealistic and rigid expectations of herself, to correct her distorted self-image, and to provide a relationship in which she felt valued and respected. We talked about how she was still mourning the absence of her father and mother in her life and how her obsession with perfection was both her way of being in control and her way of attempting to be "good enough" so that she did not lose the people she loved.

When Mary would compare herself to her peers, I placed her stress in context by reminding her of her extraordinary circumstances: balancing the roles of student, mother, and wife. I challenged Mary's distorted self-image by pointing out how her behaviors and accomplishments contradicted her perceptions of herself as incapable and defective. She was anxious about failing in school but was making As and Bs. She feared she was a bad parent but was consistent and loving with her children and always present at school, medical appointments, and extracurricular activities.

Mary was particularly concerned about her daughter, who was having academic problems and pushing the limits by challenging Mary at home. As we discussed strategies for how to respond to her daughter, we talked about her tendency to go it alone and explored how she might involve her husband more as a parent. I also shared that, having raised a daughter myself, I understood how difficult the preteen years could be. Self-disclosures like these were important to our connection and working relationship because they helped Mary feel that she was not so different or deficient.

I also made it a point to own my mistakes in the treatment. One week I missed responding to a call from Mary when she was in some difficulty. At the next session, I apologized and expressed concern that I was not there for her at a time that she needed me. After some discussion, Mary said that she appreciated this disclosure because it made her feel that I cared for her as something more than a patient.

By the end of treatment, Mary was more forgiving and accepting of herself, had begun the process of prioritizing her own needs, and acknowledged her capabilities by articulating her skills and talents as she prepared for the work world.

CONCLUSIONS

Models of adult development and research on the lives of successful women (e.g., Alfred, 2001; Lustgarten, 2008) have demonstrated the potential for life-changing transformations in the later years. In my life, these years have been the most fulfilling professionally, because my liberation from dependence on the rules and authority of external experts has allowed me to emerge secure in my own wisdom and to be directed by my "inner" voice. This does not mean that I have rejected all that I have been taught but rather that I am more discerning, integrating my truths with knowledge gleaned from others.

Lessons and Lifelines

The particular course of my professional journey was essential in my development as a clinician. The period of self-doubt, when I allowed my voice to be silenced while privileging the knowledge of others, exposed me firsthand to the pain of marginalization and oppression. This lived experience allows me to understand and empathize with my clients, who come to treatment with lives damaged from the abuse and oppression by significant others.

My lifelines during this difficult phase in my development were self-initiated activities to maintain ties to my cultural heritage and native knowledge. In my work I attempt to create lifelines for my clients by connecting them with their subjective truths and being a source of support and validation for their emerging insights. I can be optimistic about change and the potential for positive growth, and I hold this optimism for my clients, because of my own affirming life experiences.

For Future Generations

In considering the implications of my experience, one question that comes to mind is how might this path be made easier for future generations.

Given the centrality of connection and relationship in women's lives, a mentor can be an important resource, facilitating professional development. Mentoring serves multiple functions, including modeling, guidance, support, sponsorship, coaching, and confirmation (Boice, 1989; Gilbert & Rossman, 1992).

Women of color, faced with the challenges of racism and sexism coupled with the anxieties and uncertainties that effect any developing professional, may be particularly vulnerable to self-doubt and confusion about their place and about opportunities in the professional arena. They need others whom they respect and trust to acknowledge and affirm their realities to advocate for them and to support them in optimizing their strengths and capacities. Having her own lived experience, another woman of color who has successfully navigated the challenges of the professional world would be the ideal mentor—but these women are still only sparsely represented in the field. White professional women can also be valuable supports to women of color by sharing their knowledge, expertise, and experience in surviving and thriving in academia and the work world. Mentors for women of color who are developing professionals must strive to be one of those "safe spaces" where these women can come for mirroring, rejuvenation, and nurturing. Directing and connecting these women to other validating and affirming resources in the profession and larger community can also ease their learning and growing process.

If our learning and work environments were more inclusive and inviting of multiple perspectives and diverse ways of knowing, women could expend less energy in fighting to be acknowledged and recognized and would be more productive in their respective fields. As women, we must advocate for equality in the workplace and the academy. We must be visible and vocal, as leaders and teachers, and stand up for the rights of women to be heard and respected. In her work on women leaders, Lustgarten (2008) suggests many women feel that they must relinquish their feminine voice and be like men to be competitive. Little progress will be made in alleviating the oppression of women if we compromise our values to accommodate to male-dominated systems. We must demonstrate that we can achieve, and be powerful, and still be connected and caring, that we can be giving and compassionate without being self-sacrificing. We must dare to be ourselves for the sake of those coming after us.

REFERENCES

Alfred, M. V. (2001). Expanding theories of career development: Adding the voices of African American women in the White academy. *Adult Education Quarterly*, *51*, 108–127.

Black, L., & Magnuson, S. (2005). Women of spirit: Leaders in the counseling profession. *Journal of Counseling and Development, 83*, 337–342.

Boice, R. (1989). Psychologists as faculty developers. *Professional Psychology: Research and Practice, 20,* 97–104.

Bryant, R. M., Coker, A. D., Durodoye, B. A., McCollum, V. J., Pack-Brown, S. P., Constantine, M., et al. (2005). Having our say: African American women, diversity and counseling. *Journal of Counseling and Development, 83,* 313–319.

Cavanaugh, J. C., & Blanchard-Fields, F. (2002). *Adult development and aging.* Belmont, CA: Wadsworth.

Colarusso, C. A., & Nemiroff, R. A. (1981). *Adult development: A new dimension in psychodynamic theory and practice.* New York: Plenum.

Erikson, E. H. (1950).*Childhood and society.* New York: Norton.

Gilbert, L. A., & Rossman, K. M. (1992). Gender and the mentoring process for women: Implications for professional development. *Professional Psychology: Research and Practice, 23,* 233–238.

Gilligan, C. (1982). *In a different voice: Psychological theory and women's development.* Cambridge, MA: Harvard University Press.

Grier, W., & Cobbs, P. (1968). *Black rage.* New York: Basic Books.

Hooks, B. (1989). *Talking back: Thinking feminist, thinking black.* Boston, MA: South End Press.

Josselson, R. (1978). *Finding herself: Pathways to identity development in women.* San Francisco, CA: Jossey-Bass.

Levinson, D. J. (1978). *Seasons of a man's life.* New York: Knopf.

Lippert, L. (1997). Women at midlife: Implications for theories on women's adult development. *Journal of Counseling and Development, 76,* 16–22.

Lustgarten, R. (2008). Creativity, longevity and wisdom: Women's wisdom in leadership. In D. Tower, V. M. Bentz, & K. Rogers (Eds.), *Creative longevity: Essays on aging and wisdom* (pp. 55–68). Santa Barbara, CA: Fielding Graduate University.

Pargament, K. (2007). *Spiritually integrated psychotherapy.* New York: Guilford Press.

Pedersen, P. B. (1999). *Multiculturalism as a fourth force.* Philadelphia: Brunner/Mazel.

Ridley, C. R. (2004). *Overcoming unintentional racism in counseling and therapy.* Thousand Oaks, CA: Sage Development.

Scheurich, J. J. (1993). Toward a White discourse on White racism. *Educational Researcher, 22,* 5–10.

Settlage, F., Curtis, J., Lozoff, M., Silberschatz, G., & Simburg, E. J. (1986). Conceptualizing adult development. *Journal of the American Psychoanalytic Association, 36,* 347–369.

Souto-Manning, M., & Ray, N. (2007). Beyond survival in the ivory tower: Black and brown women's living narratives. *Equity and Excellence in Education, 40,* 280–290.

Vaillant, G. (2008). Does wisdom increase with age? In D. Tower, V. M. Bentz, & K. Rogers (Eds.), *Creative longevity: Essays on aging and wisdom* (pp. 1–8). Santa Barbara, CA: Fielding Graduate University.

Leaving Analysis and Moving Beyond Pain

HELENE MOGLEN

University of California, Santa Cruz, California

SHEILA NAMIR

Private Practice, Santa Cruz, California

As an analyst and an analysand, we explore reasons for not *"doing" psychoanalysis in the last third of life when our own experience became sufficiently intense to make self-exploration through pain undesirable. For the analyst, self-knowledge was inseparable from the therapeutic process: she discovered and created her selves in therapeutic relationships, which meant living in the pain of others. The analysand needed to know whether she could reinvent her life, after one of its lengthiest and most complex phases had ended. The analyst decided to turn away from a primary focus on the therapeutic other in order to commit herself to being alive with more pleasure. The analysand decided that she did not need to go back in order to move forward. For both, it was the formation of a new relationship in the last third of life that created the environment for mutual recognition and libratory self-discovery.*

. . . the analysis comes to an end because life takes on a new intensity.

(Frances Roustang, 1996, p. 113)

When we were invited to consider the topic "women doing therapy in the last third of life," we decided to turn its apparent assumption upside down. Drawing on our own experiences—which, while different therapeutically, are personally linked—we decided to consider why individuals might choose not to "do" therapy as they age. In the brief personal reflections that follow,

each of us considers her own complicated relation to psychotherapy—
Helene as analysand and Sheila as analyst. Then, in our concluding comments, we explore some of the implications of our narratives for a critique
of psychoanalysis in the context of aging.

LEAVING ANALYSIS

I have taught and written about psychoanalytic theory and have used the
interpretive strategies of psychoanalysis to read texts and to construct narratives about my life. Still, I resisted the role of analysand until my psychic
survival seemed to depend on my willingness to accept it.

In March 2000, my husband was diagnosed with a fatal brain tumor. By
July, I was living in the two-dimensional space of a continuous present,
which was suffused by images and affects of an undifferentiated past.
Memory blurred; taste vanished. I could not grasp who I was alone, nor
could I imagine who, once abandoned, I might become. During 44 years
of marriage, as our differences from one another increased, our identities
had become more entangled, like plant roots that have outgrown their origi-
nal, small pot. By the time I entered therapy, my husband was dying and the
processes of separation and psychic erasure had simultaneously begun.

Therapy provided a transitional space in which I could plumb the
depths of the past and begin to imagine a future. Through the transference,
I encountered aspects of myself that had been, over time, submerged. A new
sense of capacious multiplicity made me feel that, although I had never
known myself so little, I had never inhabited so fully the person I had
become. Both strange and familiar, mine was an uncanny self that had
survived the losses by which it had irrevocably been stamped.

As I separated the roots of the hybrid entity that my husband and I had
created, I was able to ask what I would lose with the death of the other—and
also how I might change. There was freedom in differentiation and the end
of dependency, it is true, but through the transference, vestigial relational
patterns were also reintroduced. Reenacting the role of the other, my analyst
sometimes extended forms of recognition that I identified with the good
mother; at other times, he seemed to reproduce the bad mother's imper-
viousness. Mirroring, he threatened the absence of substance. Listening
silently, he seemed not to hear.

Of course, these good and bad maternal figures were projections on the
walls of therapy's hall of mirrors, as was the analyst's construction of me as a
loquacious version of his own suffering and silent mother. Increasingly, the
theme of my analytic sessions became denial and withdrawal. I lined up my
mother, my husband, and my analyst for a target practice that was never
satisfying and that always required repetition. I knew there was another
space, inhabited by different characters, outside the mirrored hall. There

was a door, which could easily be opened, and a labyrinthine path, along which I could try to find my way.

My decision to walk through that door was prompted by a desire to redefine my relation to the other as a living presence, not as a function, a representation, or a haunting ghost. That decision was also fueled by a wish to replace self-obsession with self-expression. It was supported by my growing sense of a future that could provide alternatives to the reiterated dysfunctions of the past. Above all, I was prompted by having fallen, unexpectedly, in love.

In an intimate relationship formed in the last third of life, one's perspective is likely to be different from perspectives that governed self-perception in young adulthood and in middle age. To perceive oneself through the eyes of a loving other—another whom one had not known before—is to see oneself with startling clarity in the present. And to be recognized at that moment by the other is a validation of one's right to be whomever one has become.

The emergence in therapy of dissociated self-states had broadened the psychic repertoire that was available for enactment within the transference. Once outside the hall of mirrors I could explore those liberated, if truncated, selves more creatively in the context of this new and intense relationship. More, because my lover was another woman, substantially younger than I, the repertoire of possibilities that had been extended in analysis proved inadequate in surprising ways. Gender, age, and sexuality lost their conventional references altogether, and in order to comprehend their current meanings, I had to disinter curtailed identifications, buried memories, and transgressive desires.

If my experience as a teacher and an interpreter of literary texts had prepared me for the shifting projections and identifications of the transference, the transference served as preface to the provocative disorder of identities that I suddenly encountered. The psychic capaciousness I had enjoyed in analysis yielded to a riotous multiplicity of nascent, emergent, and developing selves that bemused but also delighted me. Male/female, mother/daughter, straight/gay, young/old, lover/friend were the more familiar binaries that were subject to experiential deconstruction. The apparent abstraction of other oppositional formulations—theory/experience, desire/identification, social/psychological, essential/relative—simply supplied more grist for the mill. None of the categories held: all were in movement and that movement signaled psychic (and also intellectual) growth. The fact that multiplicity did not become chaos had much to do with my secure position in life and with the many complicated roles I had played as I matured and aged.

Perhaps, at least initially, it was the body that provided the third term, which unlocked oppositional differences. Sex produces its own form of truth in the primal experience of the erotic. It is a truth that lies outside of language. It is fused with affectivity and is distanced from social constructions. It is attentive to the profound experience of loss, to the voiceless cries of trauma, and to the inarticulate yearnings of desire. It is enabled by empathic connection and it relies, above all, on trust. The knowledge that our bodies discovered made contradiction irrelevant. It became the bedrock on which our relationship rested.

Of course, analysts and analysands often struggle to reach that place beneath and outside of words. (It is a focus of my partner's own psychoanalytic practice.) But the route is lengthy and circuitous, and it is oriented to the past. Although the analytic relation facilitates the journey, it also provides—through its multiple projections and repetitions—its limiting conditions. The door of the hall remains to be opened; the liberating third has still to be discovered. The leap of faith must always be made. But the most important difference may be this: unlike the intensities of the erotic connection, in the regressive stage of the analytic process, pain is not bonded to pleasure.

When I left analysis, I rejected the continuous immersion in feeling and the excitement provided by the constant interrogation of self. With that decision, I also turned away from the dark insights of a sustained analytic regression. There was much in therapy that was thrilling and there was much, therefore, to be lost. But in the last third of life, time matters, and faith in the future is as important as it is rare. Pleasure and desire can no longer be taken for granted, and one is unaccustomed to bodily knowledge that actually heals. I left analysis in order to take up my life. I committed myself once again to the social, and I expanded my understanding of what it means to love.

MOVING PAST PAIN

For 40 years I traveled the landscape of therapy—being in therapy, studying to be a therapist, and practicing therapy and psychoanalysis. For most of these years, doing therapy made me feel that life was intense, magical, and meaningful. As a child, I discovered that I could survive and create meaning by helping others and that I could reside in fantasy and imagination through my connection to words and by loving. When I learned as a young adult that I could study and work from these same powerful places, I felt that I had been given a privilege and a gift. It is not surprising, therefore, that it has taken me seven years to understand why I do not want to live any longer in the lands of psychotherapy, do not want to dedicate the rest of my life to these most extraordinary and intense endeavors, and especially do not want to die in my consulting room chair. Writing this paper turns out to be part of my termination phase with psychoanalytic practice.

What does it mean to "not do" psychotherapy as a psychotherapist at this stage of life? As I seek to understand why practicing psychotherapy no longer engages me as it did for so many years, and why I have spent the last seven years disengaging from it, I begin by reviewing what it is *not*. Most published papers about changing or terminating one's psychoanalytic practice reflect on geographic moves, illness, or death. These are *not* my reasons. Nor do I think I would be considered an "aging analyst," (Tallmer, 1992) particularly in the light of papers recently published by an octogenarian and a nonagenarian about their continuing commitment to their work (Bolgar, 2002; Sanville, 2002). On many levels, my interest has not flagged. I still do derive immense pleasure from helping others come more fully alive, from hearing their life stories, from participating in the creation of their insights and collaborating in their emotional change. Creating meaning from primal feelings and preverbal states still fascinates me. Most of all, my curiosity about psychic processes and phenomena continues to be prodigious.

I was always drawn, because of my own history, to working with people at the extreme edges of being. The reasons, of course, are in my own story, and my own story determined the ways I practiced therapy and psychoanalysis. For me, the traumata before speech, the ways that memories live in the body and erupt in somatic expressions, and the silences of relationships that confuse and confound the making of meaning: these have always captured my mind and attention. Early in my life, I was one of those who did not assume that being born gave me the right to exist. Instead, doing and giving was my passport to being. I suspect that my motivations for becoming an analyst are deeply related to this lack of existential entitlement and to my discovery at age three that I would not only have to take care of myself but that I would also have to take care of my sisters. That was when my identity and career as a "compulsive caregiver" (Bowlby, 1980) began. My subsequent decision to become a psychologist, and then a psychoanalyst, felt congruent with the ways I formed attachments and with what I felt I had to offer in relationships. My identity in these roles was always subsumed under my identity as a compulsive caregiver. The existential pain and doubt that haunted me since childhood made concerns about human suffering and the desire to help those who suffered my reasons for being. From isolation and aloneness I created a life of meaning that involved my immersion in the intensity of pain. The struggle to understand both myself and others became inseparable from the therapeutic process.

This meant that living intensely and centrally in my own internal world included the internal worlds of my patients. The cocoon of psychic reality was necessary and sufficient for many years. Helping others to go inside and explore, despite their fears that they would find nothing but emptiness within, fueled my work as a therapist. Despite the primal feelings and anxieties it evoked, this experience was safer and more satisfying for me than living in the world.

Eventually, I began to feel constrained by self-awareness and self-absorption as well as by diverse transference-countertransference interplays with people who were suffering. Practicing psychotherapy, a *private* practice, creates its own isolative conundrum. Living in these dyadic relationships left me without energy and interest in larger worlds. Some years ago I wrote prophetically on a slip of paper: "The hallmark of success in my analysis is that I no longer want to be an analyst. I no longer have the passion or the need to practice a profession of self-cure."

And then, seven years ago, as I was remodeling my house in Los Angeles, opening up space so that my cozy, domestic cocoon might accommodate others, I met someone who made me want to leave the cocoon in shreds. As I realized that I was struggling more each week to return to the somber and serious world of my practice I began to understand that I did not want to live inside the pain of patients anymore, that I did not want much of my psychic and physical life to be a container for the suffering of others. What had always been a refuge and a sacred place that gave meaning to life had become a prison of pain.

I turned 50 during this awakening and felt strongly that I had done everything I needed to do, and now was free to do as I liked. My insight was not about particular patients or institutes; it was about the profession of psychoanalysis. It was inseparable from a shifting perspective on the possibilities and limitations of this last third of life.

It is not that I expect to live the last third of my life without pain—I just don't want to work within pain on an hourly, daily basis. And it is not that I expect a life of passion and intensity (which I both continue to value and to have) to be without pain, but the context for that pain and its expressions are what I now feel free to choose and create.

For me, not doing psychotherapy in the last third of life has to do with the desire for freedom—freedom from frequent suffering, from compulsive caregiving, from the need to be inside in order to feel safe. It also means freedom from seeking a cure for the suffering and pain that is inevitably reproduced by psychoanalysis itself. Now that I am living my own life more fully, freedom means no longer needing to deliver people into their lives. It means not moving to a rhythm created by the needs, demands, and limiting schedules of others, in a space that is created by many relationships lived inside a frame. Not doing psychotherapy is breaking out into the space beyond trauma, transgressing trauma's barrier. It is to break free of the constraint and restraints of my past along with its existential despairs.

My increasing interest in the world—including the ways in which psychoanalytic perspectives and theories may inform political and social life—certainly contributes to my movement away from individual psychotherapy. But mostly, and foremost, it is the desire to feel and trust the aliveness of love to the same extent that I have felt and trusted the aliveness of pain. It is a desire to live much more in pleasure.

CONCLUSION

Placing our stories in conversation with one another, we find differences between them in substance and perspective as well as a number of important assumptions that are shared. Above all, we assume that psychic growth is possible in the last third of life, and we struggle to define—in the context of our own experiences—the determining conditions of such alterations. And although each of us, in her own way, is committed to the magic and mystery of psychoanalysis, we consider how its practices can limit as well as advance psychic growth.

In addressing the possibilities and restrictions of therapeutic practice, we both inadvertently employ a series of binary oppositions in the construction of our arguments. Implicitly, we assume a distinction between psychoanalysis and a fully realized life. From this importantly weighted opposition, all the others, similarly weighted, follow: pain versus pleasure, past versus future, repetition versus innovation, the projected versus the intrinsic other, and the intrapsychic versus the social and political. As always, the oppositional structure suggests an affective intensity that signals special pleading. It is through our use of binaries, after all, that we normalize our uncommon choices, which are not often available to people in the last phases of their lives. Although our rhetorical strategy is useful, therefore, it is also decidedly misleading.

Still, despite the notes of advocacy that our narratives sound, they do point beyond the personal and eccentric to suggest how aging can be compatible with psychic growth. To the extent that we successfully make this case, we interrogate the extensive scholarly literature that identifies ageing with conservatism. We also implicitly challenge Freud, who was himself skeptical about the psychic agility of people over 50. In his essay "On Psychotherapy" (1905), Freud observes that it would be foolhardy for "old" people to undertake psychoanalytic treatment.

> The age of patients has this much importance in determining their fitness for psycho-analytic treatment, that, on the one hand, near or above the age of fifty the elasticity of the mental processes, on which the treatment depends, is as a rule lacking—old people are no longer educable—and, on the other hand, the mass of material to be dealt with would prolong the duration of the treatment indefinitely. (p. 264)

Certainly, one of our assumptions in writing our essay (and we believe it to be an assumption that is widely shared) is that older people are not only capable of psychic growth but that they may have fewer stakes in fetishizing anachronistic identities as they age. Furthermore, as our discussions of analytic strategies suggest, the amount of material that one brings into therapy does not necessarily change the length of one's analysis; it can simply provide a larger canvas on which the repetitious structures of the transference/countertransference can be played out.

Perhaps what is most significant in our stories is that both of us were open to psychic transformation when we met—and that psychoanalysis had much to do with our particular forms of readiness. Helene had been motivated to "do" therapy so that she could imagine a future that would be different from her past. In building an extension of her house, Sheila was enacting the psychic expansion, which years of "doing" therapy had made possible. The relationship we "found" together filled the space, which each of us had cleared in therapy, for psychic and social innovation. And while our readiness may have also marked the continuation of progressive ideological strains that had characterized our earlier lives, it signaled an informed desire to give progressivism a more intimate, relational meaning.

Freud was 49 when he wrote his pessimistic essay about the limitations of the aging mind. He lived for 34 more years, years in which he was extraordinarily productive. In his case, the evidence of his life refuted a theory that was apparently rooted in anticipatory dread. It is for this reason that his narrative can be read as a cautionary tale. We dread aging—not least of all, as prelude to our deaths. But it can be as rich, as complicated, as psychically transformational a phase as any that has preceded it. Openness, it turns out, is all.

REFERENCES

Bolgar, H. (2002). When the glass is full. *Psychoanalytic Inquiry, 22*, 640–651.

Bowlby, J. (1980). *Attachment and loss, volume III: Loss, sadness and depression.* London: The Hogarth Press and The Institute of Psycho-Analysis.

Freud, S. (1905). On psychotherapy. In *The standard edition of the complete psychological works of Freud* (vol. VII). (pp. 255–268). London: Hogarth Press.

Roustang, F. (1996). *How to make a paranoid laugh or, what is psychoanalysis?* Philadelphia: University of Pennsylvania Press.

Sanville, J. B. (2002). When therapist and patient are both in Erikson's eighth stage. *Psychoanalytic Inquiry, 22*, 626–639.

Tallmer, M. (1992). The aging analyst. *Psychoanalytic Review, 79*, 391–404.

"Be Kind, for Everyone You Meet is Fighting a Great Battle"

LAURA MASON

University of California–Berkeley, Berkeley, California

The longer I have lived and worked, the more complicated my view is of human suffering, of what causes psychological problems, and of what is needed to help people heal. Psychotherapists have less autonomy now than we did 25 years ago because mental health services are more regulated by managed care. Although the increased accountability is a crucial benefit for client care, the emphasis on symptom relief can be a disservice. Certainly there are some identifiable symptoms that can be extinguished, but often the wounds of life include grief, loss, relationship traumas, and other kinds of pain. Sometimes the limits of change and the pain that is part of life must be accepted. I have been influenced by experiences in rural Africa and in underserved communities in the United States about the value of social and cultural factors in psychotherapy relationships as well.

On a Thursday morning recently, my 9:00 a.m. appointment was with a woman I'd seen eight years earlier. She was returning to treatment after her mother's death. In the course of the session, this woman described a new medical symptom of her own. Her neurologist was pretty certain of the diagnosis; while not life threatening, my patient would have to choose between no longer driving and taking a strong medication. She went on to talk about her own 60th birthday, her thinning hair, and her bittersweet response to her daughter's marriage. Looking back on her own life, she recalled getting up the nerve, in 1970, to tell her father over the phone that she planned to move in with her fiancé. Her father had said to her, "We can't talk about such a thing over the company telephone! I'll call you right back." Both of us smiled with the awareness of how much things have changed since then. I thought to myself that this would be a charming story to tell her children if they ever wanted to record their mother's life story. Suddenly I realized that recording someone's life story is something that children do when their parents are older. Why was I thinking this about a woman my age?

Everything about this session reminds me that I am no longer young, nor are many of my clients. I have been a psychologist in private practice for nearly 30 years now. My practice is a general one; I do not specialize in a particular age group, diagnostic group, set of issues, or therapeutic technique. For the past 20 years, I have also worked as the clinical director of a community clinic which is staffed by doctoral students in UC–Berkeley's Clinical Science Program.

As I think back over my career and think ahead to the years that are left, there are certain trends and developments that strike me. When I entered this profession, I thought of becoming a psychoanalyst as the highest achievement I could attain. Psychoanalytic theory is still my clinical foundation, but my own personal development has led me, to my surprise, to include work in the public health arena as well. The basic unifying themes over the years, however, can be seen in my orientation toward human relationships and community contexts.

THE CHANGING LANDSCAPE OF CLINICAL PRACTICE

When I started out in private practice, the world of the clinician was much more autonomous. For clients who had health insurance, there were no session limits or eligibility requirements. There was no managed care, and there were few mandated reporting laws. Today, our profession is highly regulated. I value some aspects of this current climate: the rigorous standards of care and the attention to the rights of clients come to mind. But I deplore what I feel are the narrow definitions of "evidence-based treatments" and "medical necessity" that mark clinical psychology's pedagogy today.

In contrast to the current climate, I am much more focused now on psychotherapy as essentially a human encounter. I am particularly moved by the relational aspects of psychotherapy and by the potential for modulating and regulating intense affective states through the therapeutic relationship (see Fosha, 2000; Wallin, 2007). I think much less about my own theoretical orientation and much less about applying the correct technique than I did years ago. I place much more emphasis on the particular person with whom I am working and the particular kind of relationship, needs, and formulation that fits this individual.

When I teach my beginning graduate students about different psychotherapy theories and about the issues in evaluating the evidence for each of them, I always remind them of the famous Buddhist parable in which a king asks a group of blind men to examine and describe an elephant. Of course, each man's report depends on the part of the elephant he explored. Similarly, our theories about psychotherapy and psychopathology depend on the particular phenomenon and methodology chosen. I remember my mentor, Dr. Hilde Burton, telling me when I was a graduate student that our clinical theories are only maps. There are many different kinds of maps that are useful when undertaking a journey to an unknown place: contour maps, road maps, satellite maps. I find myself, at this time in my life, in a fairly ecumenical frame of mind; there are many kinds of maps that are useful, and what is most important to me is that our clinical theories are not the same as the phenomenon itself, any more than reading a map is the same as walking through a landscape.

THE TIME OF MY OWN JOURNEY

My sense of the immediacy and import of the experience of walking through a landscape may derive from the time in history that I came of age and the fact that my own life's journey led me through many different terrains. I started college in the 1960s and was a passionate participant in the movements of that decade: the Free Speech Movement, the Civil Rights Movement, the Anti-War Movement, and the Women's Movement. Like many young people at that time, I threw myself into alternative life choices. By the time I finished my PhD and entered the profession of psychology in 1985, I had worked as a waitress, a cross country truck driver, a dockworker, a farm worker, and on many assembly lines. I had been in and out of college over a period of 19 years, and was in my third marriage. More importantly, and more difficult for me to come to terms with personally, were the experiences I had in my family of origin with severe mental illness (Mason, 2008). My life has taught me that the place to start in any human interaction is with the person who sits before you, not any theory no matter how empirically supported.

OPENING UP TO EMOTIONAL EXPERIENCE

This point of view was not explicit when I began working as a psychotherapist, of course. When I was first in training, I worked with a woman who was 76 years of age, who had been referred by her physician for depression. Everything she talked about led back to her ex-husband's sudden request for a divorce when she was 50. Her grown children were sick of her being stuck on this event, and I too wondered why she was so preoccupied with something that had taken place over 25 years earlier. As a budding clinician and as a young person, I had implicit ideas and opinions about what it meant to be healthy and what it meant to be "stuck" in psychopathology. I don't think I was impatient or unkind toward this woman, but I do think that I approached her with an attitude that could be phrased as, "What is wrong with this woman that she hasn't moved on with her life?"

Today I think differently. I know now how adult life can be forever marked by single, profound events, particularly losses. I think that this woman's ability to lead the rest of her life is a kind of victory: she entered the work force in her fifties, maintained her own home, and had friends. With respect to those aspects of life, she wasn't "stuck" on the breakup of her marriage. She did need to talk about her divorce more than she had been able to, and the fact that she could talk about it with me was valuable to her, and powerful. As a young clinician, my unconscious goal for her was probably that she should have remarried. Today the prominent question on my mind would be, "How can I help this woman truly talk about and thereby perhaps grieve or accept what she has lost?"

CONNECTION RATHER THAN CAUSES

The first question, "What is wrong with this woman that she hasn't moved on with her life?" too easily leads to judgment and blame, to a search for causes that have the quality of determining who or what is at fault: "Who did the wrong thing?" or What cognitive distortions is she clinging to?" Although I think this line of inquiry is important, it leaves me dissatisfied as a starting point, for a number of reasons. First, it can be too easy as a clinician to distance oneself from the suffering of one's clients when one's approach is to ferret out the symptoms of the "disorder." Certainly we want to identify symptoms and make careful diagnoses, but in the context of a whole person with whom we are interacting. Second, the search for what is "wrong" can all too often take both therapist and client out of the consulting room and into what can be a dry, intellectualized world where we construct a story about past patterns, causes, and/or evidence for or against a thought.

The question, "How can I help this woman truly talk about and thereby perhaps grieve or accept what she has lost?" opens up emotional possibilities for both therapist and client. This stance begins with creating the safety within the consulting room to say and feel what is rather than moving quickly to identify and fix a problem. I think of it as entering the world of the client, however distorted, terrible, or painful. Theoretically, this evokes the work of Kohut (1984) or Schwaber (1981), who describe this phenomenon as "experience near" listening. The attachment theory based psychotherapies of Fosha (2000), Johnson (2004), and Wallin (2007) are also relevant to me, where great weight is placed on the experience of powerful, warded off affects within the safety of the therapeutic relationship. From this shared space of suffering and understanding, client and clinician can discover what ways each individual client can move through, accept, let go of, or refute that suffering.

It is at this point, however long it takes, that the time is most fruitful for working on the ways that the client has contributed to the maintenance or creation of their troubles. (This is the question that my younger self asked as "What is wrong with this woman that she hasn't moved on with her life?") Clearly, this puts me at odds with the requirements of managed health care and contemporary health care delivery, but I am encouraged by modern medical school education that underscores the relationship between physician and patient and that teaches physicians the importance of listening to their patient's stories (Fadiman, 1997; Yedidia et al., 2003). It is not surprising to me that research on patient adherence to treatment recommendations shows that adherence increases when the relationship between practitioner and client is strong (Fuertes, Boylan & Fontanella, 2009).

LOOKING FORWARD AS WELL AS LOOKING BACK

Another shift I have noticed in my clinical work as I move through middle age is one that may seem counterintuitive. Although I listen to causes and dynamics from the past in order to understand my clients' lives, I use my understanding of the past to look toward the future. How can we use our discovery of what has been missed or wounded to create what we need in the time we have left to live?

In a recent session, a woman of 50 wondered if perhaps some piece of adolescent development had been neglected in her life. She came to see me just a few months ago, initially for a consultation about her oldest daughter's inability to "move on with her life." My client described her daughter's failure to take up the tasks of becoming independent, getting up every day and brushing her teeth, going to school, tolerating the everyday tasks that we all must endure. My client has trouble with these things, too. She often finds herself moping about in the middle of the day, doing crossword puzzles online at work, procrastinating, never having really decided on a career. It is at this moment that she asks me if perhaps some piece of her adolescent development was never completed.

And it is at this moment that I find myself at one of those forks in the road that is so familiar to a clinician. I could follow the path that says that yes, she may very well have missed a piece of development as a young adult—and in fact, I think this may be true. I know that there is much to say about the ways that her mother criticized her for being unfocused, that her older sister was the competent, successful one, and so on. But the other path, the one I chose to take, was the following: "I think everyone's life has pieces that were missed or not filled out, so that we all come to whatever age we are with imbalances, development that needs to take place. What seems important right now is that this is the time in your life when you want to take up the task of being more conscious of making choices, using your time well, learning to impose structure on yourself."

Perhaps my choice in this encounter was based on my intuition that this mother was anxious about being the cause of her daughter's problems. Psychotherapy is like a chess game in these instances, because, of course, this mother needs to consider the ways that her dynamics have affected her daughter. At the same time, it would take several moves through our interaction before this woman could feel safe enough with me to look at herself and then fully think about this issue.

My rationale for taking the time to go through these moves is the value I place on kindness (Buechler, 2004). Life is hard, and people who seek treatment are in pain. It is more important to me to operate from a place of compassion and kindness than from a place of accurate interpretation (Winnicott, 1994). From the vantage point at which I sit now, I try to bring to my work the words of Philo of Alexandria: "Be kind, for everyone you meet is fighting a great battle."

As my client described the conversations between herself and her daughter, it sounded to me like the daughter might have a thought disorder and some kind of psychotic process. As subsequent evaluations bore this out, this woman stayed in treatment with me and struggled to come to terms with her daughter's illness. What anguish for a parent.

My client does not know that I have two sisters with psychotic illnesses. She does not know that I have witnessed and experienced the devastation these illnesses wreak on a family, nor does she know that my own mother has never recovered emotionally from the blame that my profession put on my mother for my sisters' illnesses. I have chosen not to tell my client about my own life story so that her therapy is maintained for her to come to terms with her own life story in whatever way she will. But of course my story allows me to sit with her in very particular ways.

WHERE I COME FROM, DEEP DOWN INSIDE

It has always been obvious to me that I chose the profession of clinical psychologist because of my excruciating experiences in my family of origin, but my relationship to this knowledge has been transformed over the years. As a young person, my orientation was toward proving that my parents were to blame for my sisters' illnesses. It wasn't only because that was the accepted explanation for schizophrenia during the late 1960s and early 1970s, it was also because I wanted to put blame somewhere, anywhere; I longed for a place to project and externalize my pain. I needed to feel that there were causes that could be identified so that there would be something that could be done. Now, of course, I hope that causes will be identified so that treatments can be more and more effective, but I am hopeful that we, as a field, can identify contributing factors and treatments with an attitude of respect, concern, and compassion.

What, then, does this mean as I sit with my client whose daughter is now in residential treatment as my client grapples with the inevitable feeling that it *is* something about her that has resulted in her daughter's illness? There is not a concerned parent in the world who would not ask such a question, nor could that parent be reassured by talk of genetics, gene-environment interaction, or any other explanation. I do tell this client and the others in my practice who have children with these illnesses, and those clients who themselves have severe illnesses (such as bipolar disorder or schizophrenia), that no one person, event, or gene is the cause. I also tell these clients that I know that my telling them these reassuring facts does not take away their belief that somehow, if only they had noticed something sooner, been more careful with their diet, been more structured or more permissive, done something differently, then perhaps they or their child would have been spared.

What am I offering then? A place where the agony, grief, hostility, guilt, and despair can be heard and experienced. A place where the essential humanity of the person who has these cruel illnesses can be honored. And a place where whatever kind of advocacy, services, and resources can be pooled. I have been so affected by these severe mental illnesses in my own family, and I have been so moved by my clients who struggle with these illnesses as well, but I have also been horrified by the mental health system that offers so little, that hospitalizes people briefly in order to stabilize them on medication then releases them with no follow-up or treatment, only to rehospitalize them, sometimes only a few days later. The thoughtful, decent, and competent social workers, psychological technicians, psychologists, psychiatrists, and staff who work in these institutions are helpless in the face of the limits dictated by a private health care system that is run for profit and a public health care system that is underfunded.

COMING FULL CIRCLE

So here I am, at the home stretch of my career, returning to my activist roots of the 1960s. As part of my faculty position at UC–Berkeley, I direct a community clinic where mental health services for underserved populations are a priority. In this situation, it is my responsibility to train graduate students in some of their first clinical experiences. I know that these students will learn all that they need to know about the science of clinical psychology from others in the department; I take it on myself to remind them of the human face of clinical work and suffering. I tell them that I am less concerned with what disorder a person has than I am with who the person is who has the disorder (Norcross, 2002).

I also have become a board member of my county mental health service (Alameda County Board of Mental Health, part of the Alameda County Behavioral Health Care Services). I have been impressed with the many groups within this large public urban system, but particularly resonant for me is the fact that a salaried Consumer Relations Manager works within the organization who is himself a consumer activist working for patient rights and an end to mental health stigma. This man has suffered from and battled schizophrenia since 1964 and has created a network within the county of support and services for mental health service consumers. Through my encounters with the people in this consumer movement, I have been struck over and over again that what they tell me has been helpful to them is not any particular type of therapy, but the meaningful, ongoing relationships with people who treated them as people, not as diseases, people who continued to be their providers even when they went off their medication, and people who believed in their capacity to have a life of independence and dignity (Goodwin & Jamison, 2007).

Another strand in my life, at this point, is the work and education I have begun in a remote, rural region of Tanzania. Through my enterprising youngest child and her relationship with Tanzanian immigrants in California, our family has forged a strong relationship with the community of Shirati, Tanzania. In my two journeys to this region I have had the privilege of being taken in by the people, with no sense of separation as a tourist.

Here, I have participated in what I can only call an unbroken world, a world where the divisions and distinctions I am accustomed to do not apply. People and animals live together, families are bound by complex and permanent webs, and most of the food you eat is food that you grew or killed that day. The poverty, malnutrition, and illnesses are overwhelming, yet what I have learned from this community is quite profound, for they live with an awareness and acceptance of risk, misfortune, and death that we ward off desperately.

In the United States we can minimize risk, and we can file insurance claims or lawsuits when misfortune occurs. We can deny death, try to control it, and take great steps to postpone it. There are many wonderful advances that we have made in the first world, with respect to longevity, health, physical, and material comfort. But all of this comes at a cost, when we live under the illusion that we have more control than we actually do, or if we foster the notion that when something goes wrong someone is liable. There is so much that we cannot change, and the awareness of this in the field of psychotherapy is reflected in the new wave of acceptance therapies (Lejune, 2007; Mara, 2004). This is such an important development; while it is true that our clinical intervention are about the ways in which people can change, limitations must be accepted as well. We are part of the world, subject to the laws of nature, not a species outside of those laws. After living with the people of Shirati, I try to bring this sense of belonging to an unbroken world to my clinical work back home.

REFERENCES

Buechler, S. (2004). *Clinical values: Emotions that guide psychoanalytic treatment.* Hillsdale, NJ: Analytic Press.

Fadiman, A. (1997). *The spirit catches you and you fall down.* New York: The Noonday Press.

Fosha, D. (2000). *The transforming power of affect: A model for accelerated change.* New York: Basic Books.

Fuertes, J., Boylan, L., & Fontanella, J. (2009). Behavioral indices in medical care outcome: The working alliance, adherence and related factors. *Journal of General Internal Medicine, 24*(1), 80–85.

Goodwin, F. & Jamison, K. (2007). *Manic-depressive illness: Bipolar Disorder and recurrent depression* (2nd ed.). New York: Oxford University Press.

Johnson, S. (2004). *The practice of emotionally focused couple therapy.* New York: Bruner/Routledge.

Kohut, H. (1984). *How does analysis cure?* Chicago: University of Chicago Press.

Lejeune, C. (2007). *The worry trap: How to free yourself from worry and anxiety using acceptance and commitment therapy.* Oakland, CA: New Harbinger Publications.

Marra, T. (2004). *Depressed and anxious: The dialectical behavior therapy workbook for overcoming depression and anxiety.* Oakland, CA: New Harbinger Publications.

Mason, L. (2008). My story is one of loss. In S. Hinshaw (Ed.), *Breaking the silence: Mental health professionals disclose their personal and family experiences of mental illness* (pp. 25–43). New York: Oxford University Press.

Norcross, J. (2002). *Psychotherapy relationships that work: Therapist contributions and responsiveness to patients.* New York: Oxford University Press.

Schwaber, E. (1981). Empathy: A mode of analytic listening. *Psychoanalytic Inquiry, 1*, 357–392.

Wallin, D. (2007). *Attachment in psychotherapy.* New York: Guilford.

Winnicott, D. (1994). *Holding and interpretation: Fragments of an analysis.* New York: Grove Press.

Yedidia, M., Gillespie, C., Kachur, E., Schwartz, M., Ockene, J., Chepaitis, A., Snyder, C., Larare, A., & Lipkin, M. (2003). Effect of communications training on medical student performance. *Journal of the American Medical Association, 290*(9), 1157–1165.

Losing Certainty and Finding Voice: One Therapist's Reflections on Doing Therapy in the Last Third of Life

JUDITH V. JORDAN

Jean Baker Miller Institute, Lexington, Massachusetts

In this autobiographical and personal paper, the author addresses her development of voice and confidence in a relational model of healing over a period of 35 years. Departing from the "objective" and impersonal journal style typically privileged in peer-reviewed journals, this article places the development of relationship at the center of therapeutic change. It honors the question "who tells the story and who does the telling serve?" Thus a retrospective, anecdotal, personal introduction to this author, developing this theory (Relational-Cultural Theory) is at the core. In the course of reading it, the author hopes that younger practitioners will find validation and/or inspiration to listen themselves and others into creative voice. That is another facet of working in clinical settings in the latter years: to encourage new voices, new practices, and to engender hope in the abiding resilience of the human spirit.

To write on this theme, I turned my focus on doing therapy in the last third of life. This proved to be a daunting task for me. The impulse to deny that I am indeed in the last third of my professional life is strong. Somehow, I thought, others in their 60s may be at that point, but surely I am still a young, enthusiastic practitioner, learning and charting new territory. Yes and no. I am still learning, but I am far from a young beginner. It is difficult to frame what my practice is like now without delineating the journey that got me to this place. And I clearly can no longer speak in the abstract; the language of psychological inquiry has been too often framed in the impersonal. Writing for journals, we are warned not to include the personal pronoun "I." And yet that is what being in the last third of life is so much about: acknowledging that there is not *one* truth, *one* way of doing therapy, but that all truths and therapies are contextual, historical, and ultimately personal. I am trying not to apologize for how personal my response to the "job" of writing this article is. This is part of the message about the last third of life practice.

THE PERSONAL VOICE

I welcome the opportunity to write about my journey as a therapist; I like shedding the pretense of objectivity and the mantle of "expert." Almost as far back as I can remember, I wanted to be a psychologist. My mother was always interested in psychiatry, and volumes of Freud, Menninger, and others surrounded me in my childhood home. All of my siblings went into the helping fields: my oldest sister became an Episcopalian priest (and sculptor), my brother became a psychiatrist (and businessman) and my next older sister is a practicing clinical social worker. So despite lapses in my interest in becoming a psychologist—when I wanted to be an actress, a cowboy, a physician, an artist—my interest endured and was supported in my family of origin.

I majored in psychology in college, only to decide I wanted nothing to do with the field. The psychology of my college years was about teaching albino rats to press the bar and receive pellets of food. That was not for me. Perhaps I would be an artist after all. Then, two years later, I was back in graduate school preparing to be a clinical psychologist.

Part of the fascination of psychology for me was trying to get at the meaning of life. I was always pestering people with questions about what life meant to them. I wanted to know if there was some universal reason that we were here and what kept people going through the hardships of life. Perhaps I was "old" before my time. My sister playfully sent me a T-shirt last year that had on it the message "Maybe the hoky poky *is* what it's all about."

I'm sure another part of my interest in psychology was about trying to figure out my own trajectory. What was I meant to be doing? (I kept thinking there was a big plan somewhere.) Why were girls treated differently from boys? (That was a big one for me.) Why did some kids get treated so badly in school, while others enjoyed good treatment from both teachers and peers? Why was early adolescence, with all its in-groups and out-groups, so very painful? Why did people make fun of me for being so tall and getting good grades? Why, why, why. I remember being a helper to the school psychologist in elementary school. (I thought I was being a helper, at least.) When others picked on kids, I suggested they were unhappy and "needed help" (my mothers' voice?).

I went to a graduate program in clinical psychology (Harvard) that didn't really believe in clinical psychology as a discipline, and, in fact, the program was phased out two years after I entered with a class of about eight people. The other two women in my class left at the end of the first year. I was told, by several fellow graduate students and one professor, that I was "wasting the space" that could be filled by a man who would eventually contribute something to the field, while I would likely be staying home and having babies. This was reminiscent of the advice my mother received when she applied to medical school many years (40 years, I think) before: go home, marry a nice man, and raise a family. So much for progress.

Much of our time in graduate school was spent learning to critique existing theories and being told that the only worthwhile path was to become an academic. I became a clinician. When it came time to do my dissertation, I decided to work on the experience of competence and gender. Several professors tried very hard to get me to do something "important," like a study on schizophrenia. I was told I was "throwing myself away" in my study of girls and women and in my interest in clinical work. I had received a commendation from the department for outstanding achievement, and my professional choices did not match their expectations for me. Why wasn't I following in their footsteps? For many years afterward I would get calls from former professors telling me they had just heard of a "plum" position in some university, and would I finally consider such an appointment?

I persevered in my clinical pursuits. I chose my internship based on an interview with Irene Stiver. In the room with her there was warmth, intensity, and intelligence. And I was drawn to it. But the internship I chose was pretty psychoanalytic, so I spent much of my year trying to learn how to be neutral, objective, and "nongratifying." I also spent the year being told I was "too nice" and that I probably had difficulty with my aggression. Then, when I did engage in battles over concepts like "penis envy" I was told I was "an angry woman." To many of my supervisors, my anger just proved that penis envy was real. Later, when I assumed a staff position in this same institution and I was an outspoken critic of many of the classical analytic precepts being taught there, I was treated as "a *very* angry woman."

Despite these obstacles, I found the connections with some supervisors compelling and helpful. Similarly, years later, as director of training, I found the relationships with students important as I tried to help them navigate the traditional theories and the sometimes distancing and judgmental treatment of patients.

QUESTIONING THE PREVAILING THEORIES

I never experienced a sense of absolute certainty about my clinical work, but I knew that a lot of what I'd been taught wasn't useful. And I felt that some of it was hurtful to my clients. In particular, I felt that women were misunderstood by the prevailing psychological theories. I sought others who were questioning the way therapy was being done, which at that point was a mixture of Freudian analytic and object relations approaches.

I can remember, in my training, learning to keep my mouth shut about my failure to understand some of the more complicated theories. I remember fearing that I would reveal my lack of theoretical sophistication and feeling that my ignorance would be interpreted as a sign of my "resistance" or of some irreparable personal flaw.

I felt my supervisors had X-ray vision. I felt they knew everything that was wrong with me, that they had a sure answer to each quandary I faced with uncertainty. I gave them a lot of power. Many of them comfortably accepted the power I granted.

I was young, resilient, and tried hard to be there for my patients/clients. (I could never decide on a term for the people I work with in therapy that felt "right," and I still can't.) But I often thought my supervisors would wag their fingers if they could hear the dumb things I was saying in therapy sessions. I sensed they would be critical when I could not maintain perfectly "evenly hovering attention" or "neutrality." It would be seen as a failure of my boundaries or understanding. With some good accessible supervisors, I could safely explore these questions. But with many, I felt that to do so would be opening myself to their unfriendly, pathologizing scrutiny.

I persevered. Then I found three colleagues who were similarly struggling, although at different stages in their professional careers. One was my department head, Irene Stiver, who had so impressed me in my first interview. Another was Jean Baker Miller, whose book *Toward a New Psychology of Women* published in 1976 had made such a difference to me and so many other women. The other, Janet Surrey, was a postdoc at the hospital where I was junior staff. We four began meeting and talking. We talked about our "cases," the therapy work we were doing, what felt wrong about existing understandings of women, and what felt wrong in the field of psychotherapy. We met twice a month.

CREATING A NEW MODEL

About three years after we began meeting, Jean Baker Miller became director of the Stone Center at Wellesley College. Jean suggested that we needed to start writing about the things we were talking about together. Reluctantly, some of us agreed to do this, doubting inwardly that we had anything of worth to contribute.

When Jean saw the need for us to present at professional gatherings, I was terrified. I was seriously phobic about speaking in public. In graduate school, a professor who said I had written the best comprehensive exam of any student he'd ever taught scolded me for never speaking up in class. He gave me cognitive behavioral relaxation tapes to try to help me with my "problem." (Carol Gilligan had not yet written her paper on the loss of voice in women.) Despite this history of public silence, with urging and support I agreed to give a 10-minute talk at a large gathering in Toronto. At first I had suggested that I could write the paper and Jean could deliver it. But, as Jean rightly said, "Judy, voice isn't just a metaphor.... We really do have to speak our truths!" So, reluctantly, I agreed. My colleagues would be with me, and if I fainted they could pick me up. I did not faint; I gave my short paper on empathy and the mother-daughter relationship and sat down in a pool of perspiration. A gentleman in the audience came to the microphone in the back of the room and said, "Dr. Jordan, would you care to comment on the implications of empathy for Marxist and capitalist systems of government?" I completely dissociated as I tried to decipher what he was asking. Finally I gathered my wits and said it was an interesting question and that I was sure he had some thoughts on the topic; he did, and he expounded on them for 10 minutes. I had spoken, but my fear of public speaking was abiding. Over time, with Jean and others' support, I tried again and again to find a voice, finally overcoming (for the most part) my terror.

And, over time, I began to grasp that this man's question in Toronto, which had seemed to come out of left field, actually spoke to the way that this new theory we were developing (Relational-Cultural Theory, or RCT as it's come to be known) was more than a modification of existing therapy practices (Jordan, 1997). It took a while before I grasped how revolutionary it was to try to shift the paradigm of psychology from one focused on separation (the I) to one focused on connection (the We). Such a theory shift has broad societal implications.

When Jean and the three of us began meeting, there was no big agenda to come up with a new theory. We all needed support and encouragement at our respective teaching hospitals, and we all felt the pain of being misrepresented by existing theories.

The first time Jean suggested we ought to be writing and presenting our ideas at conferences, we all felt surprised and a bit anxious. Each of us held our private worries that we were incapable of such undertakings. I remember one evening in particular where we went around the room and each of us shared our very private convictions that we were not "smart enough" to have anything to say to a larger audience. I remember the shock when I realized these esteemed colleagues of mine, who I tremendously admired, held the same doubts.

Age was a part of that shock. Irene and Jean were at least in their late 40s or early 50s. They were my mentors. Surely they had moved past whatever silencing had occurred in their respective lives. And of course they had, in many ways, in ways that became beacons for others. But they, too, were still plagued with that sense of "one day they will discover I am a fraud." I think there was a jolt for me that if we were going to take ourselves, our ideas, and our feelings seriously, we were going to have to do it together. And that's what we did. We encouraged one another and listened one another into voice. Slowly, I saw all of us grow, not in an arrogant kind of confidence but in a kind of increasing belief in the importance of the changes we were advocating.

This gradual shift, the growth of belief, which began almost 30 years ago, has been sustained and grown. I have continued for these past 30 years to learn, to grow, to doubt, to work at holding my beliefs about what the world needs and about what I have to offer.

Today, in addition to the direct therapy work I do, I also spend time writing, supervising (individually and in groups), teaching and presenting workshops, and giving conferences. I have the opportunity to interact with many different clinicians and theoreticians. I consider myself lucky to have such a large and varied group to interact with and to learn from.

One of my long-term clients commented recently:

> We've been at this, off and on, for many years. I don't know if it's just because I'm more comfortable with you, but I'd say you're pretty different now than you were when I first saw you. You seem more mellow, more real, less stiff. It's not that you talk a whole lot about your own life, but I feel like I do know you better . . . here, responding with me. Sometimes, in the early days, I felt a little hesitation when you answered one of my questions or let me see how I affected you. The flow feels less interrupted by whatever might have been going on.

I think "what was going on" was that I was checking in, mentally, with supervisors in my head, or seeking theory to get us through some difficult moment, a kind of internal voice saying "you should do this, or that wouldn't be right, or you should know more about how to respond in this moment than you do." I remember, at hard moments in therapy, wishing my supervisor Irene Stiver could be there to help me, and I remember sometimes being relieved that she wasn't there to see what a bad job I was doing.

I think this uncertainty, the doubt of "am I doing a good enough job? Am I helping enough?" is not uncommon in young therapists (though some of it might be my own struggles with a sense of competence). I hear from students (when they have the courage to tell me) how they often aren't sure they said or did the "right" thing, how sometimes, at the end of a session, they flail about, trying to find something to "give" the client in the way of an "interpretation" or a piece of wisdom to take away because they're not sure they did anything helpful in the session.

THE GIFTS OF AGING

I have continued my collaboration with valued colleagues. I have put together retirement parties and memorial services for some of them. There has been stinging sadness and aloneness in watching these friends pass away. I have experienced what people refer to as "moving up to the front lines"; mine is the next generation that will be felled. There is a loss of mothers, of those who led the way. There is a deeper appreciation of the wrenching consequences of aging and death. At times I have been embarrassed by my own hubris, as a young person who believed that I "got" what the death of a loved one was like or what it was like to get older and slower and stiffer and more tired. I did kind of "get" it, but in a more heady way. Now, when clients talk about losses and deaths, I am "with" them in a new way. I "get" their losses more deeply, as they resonate with my own increasing losses, and the impact of an aging body is no longer a hypothetical.

So, aging has deepened my appreciation for the aging of others. (I remember Irene Stiver telling me "Aging isn't for the weak." I thought I understood. I didn't really.) And aging has also given me a different understanding of youth. It has given me a more expanded sense of what the actual difficulties are in each stage of life. Sometimes, it has made me a little impatient with the worries that plague people who have the privilege of youth and much comfort. I have to work, sometimes, not to fall into a kind of bitterness or world-weary superiority, exactly what I remember as a young person I hated in older people—the "youth is wasted on the young" mentality.

Then there's the presumed understanding of what it feels like to suffer the death of people we love. When I was younger, my concern for clients going through the lingering deaths of parents, friends, partners was genuine and heartfelt, as was my experience of trauma with them when tragedy struck. I was sad, I was "with" my clients around their losses, but I now see an enormous hubris on my part, because I was someone who had suffered few personal losses. I had an intuitive sense of the pain, and I had been taught the importance of losses in people's lives, but I was probably far from grasping the complexity and emotional truth of their pain. I came to appreciate that pain more as those closest to me began to fall ill and die.

I am more patient now. Paradoxically I also experience an urgency about life that I didn't when I was younger. I feel clearer about my stance that we grow through relationships, that it is the relationship that heals people in therapy. I feel more comfortable with the intangibles about that belief—the places of not knowing quite how it all works—and still believing that it works.

I feel both the smallness and the expansiveness of the work I do. The changes we help people make are often so subtle, so minute. Sometimes even those elude us. And yet I believe that those small changes can alter the trajectory of an individuals' life in potent ways. I believe that what I learn about change, what facilitates it and what impedes it, is a crucible that I must carefully protect and carry to all those who are invested in change of any kind—social justice or personal growth.

SOCIAL RESPONSIBILITY

My sense of responsibility for the larger good grows. I try to live each day and bring to each therapy my sense that things can change for the good, despite an enlarging cloud of pessimism and cynicism that hovers over and around me and my clients. My urgency about addressing the forces of disconnection in our society remains; perhaps it has intensified. While I do not proselytize with clients, I support their engagement with others as a path of personal psychological healing and as a way toward social healing.

Perhaps with aging comes an increasing awareness of how small we are and how short our individual lives are. This does not interfere with my desire to make those small, transient lives happier and more productive for all those who I am privileged to work with (and my own as well). But it does lead to an emphasis on what does "work" for a person, where the genuine sources of joy and growth are.

It also leads to a more humble acceptance of what might not be amenable to change, even with the most Herculean effort on my part or on the part of my client. The Alcoholics Anonymous serenity prayer seems more and more wise: "Grant me the serenity to accept the things I cannot change, the courage to change those things I can, and the wisdom to know the difference." It reminds me also of another piece of wisdom, from the poet John Keats, an invitation "to explore the capacity to remain in uncertainty, mystery and doubt, without irritable reaching after fact or reason" (Keats, 1818/1987, p. 43). I think about a framed cross-stitch that hung in my family's living room: "This too shall pass away."

Harry Stack Sullivan's statement that we are all more simply human than not also serves as a guide. I feel less pressure to have "solved" all of my problems, less pressure to lead an impossibly exemplary life, and more patient with my own and others' flaws and what the British call "muddling through." I still struggle with shame, wishing my life were more tranquil or more "psychologically" or spiritually evolved, but these pressures or wishes fade more quickly.

This doesn't mean I'm at a stage of thinking that goals or intentions no longer matter. I try to bring to my practice a sense that we are all trying to live our values, to contribute to others, to heal and grow. But I am much more deeply aware of the inevitable limitations of such a process, that we are all "works in progress."

Many years ago, when we were working on our RCT model (Jordan, Kaplan, Miller, Stiver, & Surrey, 1991; Miller and Stiver, 1997), Jean Baker Miller firmly insisted we call everything we wrote a "Work in Progress." It was not, and should not be presented as, a finished "theory." Our work was constantly open to rethinking, shifting, opening new areas of "not knowing." It was to be in relationship with its creators and with its practitioners. The model itself is "in relationship," responsive, open, and evolving.

APPRECIATING THE MYSTERY

While there is more appreciation of the intangible, perhaps mysterious aspects of therapy, and an increased attitude of listening, waiting, not doing, there is also an increased sense of making use of "what works." That means, in some ways, being more eclectic, sorting out when more instrumental interventions might bring relief or movement. It also means making liberal use of consultants and referrals for CBT (cognitive-behavioral therapy) or internal family systems work or DBT (dialectical-behavior therapy) or EMDR (eye movement desensitization and reprocessing).

I guess one of the graces of growing older is realizing that life is all about learning—not knowing, not having the answers, not certain, but growing and learning and finding some graceful ways to continue on the path of being a learner, "Zen Mind; Beginners Mind," or some variation of that.

In therapy there are two fallible human beings and two wise people. Both are true. And there is such a thing as "fluid expertise," where the understanding, the growth, moves back and forth. Mostly, I feel fortunate to have entered a professional field that affords so many opportunities to learn and join others in their quest for meaning, to participate in relationships that are specifically structured to contribute to personal growth.

RELATIONAL MINDFULNESS

I increasingly bring my appreciation of meditation to my therapy work. Years ago (35, to be exact), when I first started meditating, it was considered "woo-woo," way out there, the stuff of the Beatles and other counterculture hippies. Or it was considered a sign of spiritual interest, which, at the time, in psychological circles, was often considered suspect (one step away from psychosis). I kept my zafu (cushion for meditating) in the closet of my office at the very established and proper psychiatric hospital where I worked. I would bring it out, privately, every morning before I began my work to get "clear," so that I could be more present with my clients. I originally sought training in meditation as a "stress management" program. I studied with a former social psychology professor from a Boston University. Later I was to study with a revered meditation teacher from India, Vimala Thakar, who had worked with Krishnamurti and had been involved with Gandhi's walk to the sea. She noted that both meditational presence and social action were necessary for the world to become a better place. (She didn't quite put it that way, but that's what it summed to.) I was extremely fortunate to participate in retreats with her, several times in the United States and several times in a lovely old villa in northern Italy with an international gathering. She helped me with my struggle with "ego" and "self" and provided a beacon of inspiration for my belief in the centrality of relatedness. Meditation, as I understand it, is all about being present, being in relationship.

This wealth of insight and practice was creeping, slowly and indirectly, into my theory and my clinical work. Only as I have aged have I become comfortable with the power of this work. Seeing the power of it in my own life, I am delighted to pass on this opportunity to others. Happily, accompanying my maturing comfort with this path, the world is beginning to appreciate the power of meditation in healing. There are now numerous books on using meditation in helping people with anxiety, depression, and other mental health afflictions (Begley, 2008; Teasdale et al., 2000; Goleman, 2006).

Dan Goleman, a great integrator of Western psychology and eastern meditational practices and a former science writer for the *New York Times* was a classmate of mine in clinical psychology at Harvard in the 1960s. I am grateful to him for the significant bridging he has done between these two worlds. We know now that meditation is not only good for our clients directly when they practice it, but we have data that clients of therapists who meditate gain more from therapy as well (Grepmair et al., 2007). Teasdale and colleagues (2000), following Jon Kabat-Zinn's protocol for helping people manage stress through mindfulness meditation, found that with ordinary treatment 34% of patients were free of relapse, but with mindfulness-based cognitive therapy 66% remained relapse free—a 44% reduction in the risk of relapse among those who received mindfulness based cognitive therapy.

Most recently, we have seen the beginning of a most important rapprochement between neuroscience and meditation. Some of the most compelling data supporting the usefulness of meditation comes from the world of neuroscience. In study after study, there has been support for the power of attention to change the brain (Begley, 2008). In addition to the very hopeful news about the expansive neuroplasticity of the brain, we are learning that relationships characterized by empathy and compassionate attention also powerfully alter the brain and its functioning (Goleman, 2006; Siegel, 1999). Shaver has looked at ways to enhance altruism and compassion through meditation training (Begley, 2008).

TODAY, IN MY WORK

Having been schooled to understand people as basically selfish, greedy, and motivated by self-interest, I am delighted to begin to deconstruct this negative image of myself and my fellow beings. For too long we have believed that at our core we are aggressive, self-serving, and mean, that we need to be whipped into shape by rigorous social training to overcome our innate selfishness. Now I can celebrate what we know is the natural tendency to yearn for connection, to want to contribute to the growth of others, to reach out to others for comfort and support when we feel fearful or threatened. I am happy to challenge the prevailing cultural ideals of "standing on your own"—finding courage alone, practicing independence, and denying the reality of human vulnerability, for those ideals put us at odds with our neurobiology and our biology. We need other people throughout the lifespan. We are highly interdependent creatures. Why hide our dependencies with denial, by making the network of supporting people invisible? Why pretend to be invulnerable in the face of inevitable knowledge of our mortality, our potential to be wounded? Why pretend that those who suffer pain regarding social exclusion are simply "wimps" (Eisenberger & Lieberman, 2004) rather than appreciating the very real pain that social exclusion creates for people? Why not put the energy that goes into this denial and charade into helping build supportive and growth-fostering social connections that all people can count on and contribute to?

These are the thoughts and hopes that occupy me today in my work.

Some would say I have lost my "objectivity" or become too "political." I would say that most of our so-called objectivity in the field of psychology is a myth, just as meritocracy is a myth, just as a "level playing field" is a myth. To maintain such myths is as much a political act as to challenge those myths. As my colleague Maureen Walker advises: notice who tells the story and who the telling serves. There is always bias and investment in particular stories defining what is "core" or most human.

I am becoming more comfortable with my biases, owning them, naming them, and trying to humbly accept the limitations they impose on my understandings of difference. I try to limit their negative impact on others. As much as I wish I could say I am able to simply be present, accepting, warm, and providing healing energy to the people I work with, I bring a lot of baggage to my work. Some of it I'm aware of, some of it I'm not. The best I can do is try to be responsible and responsive, to stay open. I particularly try to stay open to the ways in which I learn that I am "off," or obscuring another's truth with my own certainty, bias, or simply "not seeing."

While I am committed to helping the clients I work with feel better and be happier, I increasingly hold another, I think equally pressing, agenda. That is to help them feel more empathic and compassionate with themselves and with others. Happiness is a complex phenomenon. It can be a blip that is not easily replicated. But I believe the long-lasting release from suffering is not engendered by moments of personal happiness. I believe that lessening human suffering involves a commitment to the well-being of others, in part because we are "wired" to participate in growth-fostering relationships, not just as recipients of others' gifts to us but as mutually engaged participants. As we fully take in that our beings are "beings in relation," not "selves" standing separately and growing in isolation, we begin to see, know, and feel our ultimate interconnectedness.

THE POWER OF HOPE

I want to return to the issue of hope.

We live in a cynical time. At least in the past decade this was so. Perhaps change is finally coming in 2009? At times I have succumbed to a kind of existential lassitude or even despair. So much has looked, and unfortunately still looks, gloomy for the world: increasing disparities between the rich and the poor, hunger, global warming, wars, terrorism, new waves of mass trauma to add to the thousands of cases of personal trauma. Manipulative and cynical politicians have preyed on our fears. Where is the comfort in this world? Where is the safety to turn to others when we are afraid? In the United Sates, a country marked by great privilege, one-quarter of the people will suffer an episode of depression at some point in their lives; another one-quarter will suffer with clinical anxiety. Half the population of this affluent country will experience serious challenges to their psychological well-being.

Some have suggested that hopelessness is at the core of depression. In helplessness and hopelessness, people cease feeling that they can make a difference, that they can have an effect on either the material world or the human world; people cease feeling that they matter. As I write this I learn that New Orleans, decimated by Hurricane Katrina three short years ago, is about to be hit by Hurricane Gustav, and people are being evacuated. I recall the faces of those left behind, ignored, not responded to with Katrina, and I shudder with horror, as I do when I see the gaunt faces of children starving in third world countries and the trying-to-be-brave faces of soldiers being sent off to war.

Relational hope tells us that we can have an impact on others. We can contribute to the development of relationships that support and nourish people. We need to believe in human connectedness, that most people, at their core, do want to care and matter to one another. We yearn for connection.

A model of human experience that emphasizes our separateness works against our sense of basic connection and belonging. It creates conditions in which isolation, and resulting hopelessness and fear, thrive. Hope arises in relationship. Hope arises where change is deemed possible. Hope arises where one anticipates responsiveness and where dignity and respect prevail. Under these conditions, our neuronal pathways can shift, bringing us closer to our deep yearning for connection.

We need connection. We need to be part of something larger, beyond our small selves. We need to embrace and practice the repair of disconnection; we need to see the human condition of ultimate vulnerability as dignified and worthy of respect and care.

As a therapist, I increasingly hold the sense of possibility in relationship, the hope that where disconnections once prevailed, growth-fostering connections can take hold. While in my work I witness some of the most painful fallout from destructive relationships and misguided efforts at gaining safety through exercising limiting power over others, I must hold that thread of hope, hope of finding and providing a home in relationships that nourish us to our core, warming our hearts and changing our brains.

At the personal level, this spells the end of unending suffering. At the communal level, this offers the hope of a caring, human ark to carry us all toward healing.

REFERENCES

Begley, S. (2008). *Train your mind, change your brain*. New York: Ballantine Books.

Eisenberger, N., & Lieberman, M. (2004). Why rejection hurts: A common neural alarm system for physical and social pain. *Trends in Cognitive Science, 8,* 294–300.

Goleman, D. (2006). *Social intelligence: The new science of human relationship*. New York: Bantam Books.

Grepmair, L., Metterlehner, F., Lower, T., Bachehler, E., Rother, W., & Nickel, M. (2007). Promoting mindfulness in psychotherapists in training influences the treatment results of their patients: A randomized double blind, controlled study. *Psychosomatics, 76,* 332–338.

Jordan, J. (Ed). (1997). *Women's growth in diversity*. New York: Guilford.

Jordan, J., Kaplan, A., Miller, J., Stiver, I., & Surrey, J. (1991). *Women's growth in connection*. New York: Guilford.

Keats, J. (1818/1987). Letter to "My darling brothers." In R. Gittings (Ed.), *The letters of John Keats*, pp. 40–46. Oxford: Oxford University Press.

Miller, J., & Stiver, I. (1997).*The healing connection*. Boston: Beacon Press.

Siegel, D. (1999). *The developing mind: How relationship and the brain interact to shape who we are*. New York: Guilford Press.

Teasdale, J., Segal, Z., Williams, J., Rigeway, V., Sralsky, J., & Lau, M. (2000). Prevention of relapse in major depression by mindfulness based cognitive therapy. *Journal of Consulting and Clinical Psychiatry, 68,* 615–623.

Framing Lives: Therapy with Women of a "Certain Age"

MARY M. GERGEN

Penn State University–Brandywine

Women face powerful and negative stereotypes of who they will become as they age. They can either fight against them or they can succumb. From a social constructionist position, one may question any given formulation of reality, including the nature of aging. Because no image of aging is compulsory, there are ways of resisting the tide of negativity associated with it. Combating these negative stereotypes are the increasing numbers of older people who have greater financial resources and political influence than ever before. Enriching relationships also help undermine these stereotypes. Therapists, as relational partners, can support negative stereotypes or resist them. Working in favor of resistance is the general tendency for older people to be less emotionally labile and to be wiser than younger people in confronting adversity. Therapists also are helpful to clients facing the diverse transitional challenges of aging and in realizing aging's positive potential.

Almost 20 years ago I wrote a piece called "Finished at Forty: Women's Development Within the Patriarchy" (Gergen, 1990). I was attempting then to express my concerns about society's views of mature women, and how psychological theories, in particular, tended to support the negativity and neglect of the broader society (Gannon, 1999). Today, I would probably call the article "Finished at 50" because, to paraphrase some recent cultural mavens, 50 is the new 40. Notwithstanding this inflation in the exact age in which one is "finished," the claim I made stands: there is a dearth of psychological theories about women as older adults, except for a few descriptions of menopause, most of which are dire, followed by widowhood some decades later (Martin, 1999; Schmidt & Rubinow, 1991). Perhaps today one could add dementia, diseases, and death to the list. I think a major reason for this lack of interest in older women in psychology is that it simply mirrors the more general societal disinterest in older people, especially older women. Why is there such a negative space when there could be something more positive and profound? I would suggest it has to do with the American stereotype of aging, which tends to be a combination of undifferentiated and dysphoric images, which would discourage anyone from pursuing further inquiry, either in a social or scientific realm.

In what follows I will first explore the negative stereotypes and their negative effects. This will set the stage for considering the possibilities of transforming not only the conception of aging but the forms of life that may follow from a changed conception. Here the emphasis will be on the potentials of social construction to generate a vision of positive aging. This discussion will lead to a consideration of some major forces contributing to positive aging. I hope this discussion will furnish resources for therapists treating women, especially older ones. Finally, I will turn more directly to issues of therapy, at the paper's close. Interspersed throughout the text is a "chorus of resonant voices." Many of these voices are drawn from everyday life experiences.

THE NEGATIVE STEREOTYPES AMONG US

What is it that comes to mind when we think of an old woman? The words that spring forth are never very attractive. The images, few though they may be, are also unappealing. There is the little old lady, perhaps with tennis shoes, unfashionably dressed, unstylish grey hair, and unadorned with either makeup or jewelry. There is the "battle ax"—large, bossy, and belligerent, a la Ma Kettle of 1940's movie fame. She is a sight to behold, and her temper and obnoxious qualities precede her. There are those in wheelchairs, or, heaven forbid, behind the wheel, and those with canes, wrinkled and bent; they are to be found in nursing homes, slowly crossing streets, or in Florida, complaining that the grandchildren never call.

These negative stereotypes are deeply embedded in American culture. Long ago, Sigmund Freud (1927) had words for the differences between the sexes, even at the relatively early age of 30. "Women oppose change, receive passively, and add nothing of their own" (p. 137) he wrote in a paper titled "Some Psychological Consequences of the Anatomic Distinction Between the Sexes." He also believed that women are far more masochistic and narcissistic than men and more prone to neurosis, that they are rigid and unchangeable by the age of 30, and that they are unable to equal the high moral character of men. While Freud may be regarded as "old fashioned" and limited in his views, the tendency to equate old women with similar traits is daunting. In addition, older women are thought of as lacking in productivity, dull intellectually, perhaps even senile, and likely to be depressed (Nelson, 2002). Overall, the stereotypes of aging are more detrimental to women's standing in the world than men's, and this is particularly notable in what is considered acceptable appearance. The double standard of physical attractiveness and sex appeal allows a much greater latitude for men than for women (think Henry Kissinger versus Madelyn Albright) (Daniluk, 1998).

One of the most odious aspects of stereotyping is that those who are the focus of the image absorb its content. As one becomes conscious of a negative identity category, such as "an aging woman," one is likely to think and act in relationship to it. This tendency is called stereotype threat (Steele, 1997), and it has been shown to be a powerful influence on people's actions. Asian women who are reminded they are Asian before a math test improve their scores; Asian women reminded of their gender before the same exam do worse (Shih, Pittinsky, & Ambady, 1999). In each case, they are responding to the attributes of the stereotype. By accepting the stereotypes, racial minorities become racists; gays, homophobic; and women, sexist. Individuals become victims of their own perceptions and thus less confident of their abilities, talents, desires, and motivations when they run counter to the stereotypes. The outcome of this effect is a self-fulfilling prophecy. As we age, we begin to talk about our "senior moments," our failing memories, and our aging bodies. We judge the appropriateness of our actions by our age. We wonder if we should be seen in public in certain clothing, hairstyles, and makeup, if we should travel to certain places, buy certain cars, or dare to take up challenging tasks. Older people are also ageist.

One of the most startling pieces of research involves the impact of accepting or rejecting the negative stereotypes of aging on longevity. Researchers at Yale University's Department of Epidemiology and Public Health carried out a longitudinal study of 660 people over the age of 50. First they were asked about their agreement with the popular stereotypes that as you get older you lose your pep, things get worse, you are less useful, and you are less happy. Researchers then tracked the sample for decades. Those who disagreed with the stereotypes lived seven-and-one half years longer than those who agreed with them. This was a greater gain in longevity than that associated with low blood pressure, low cholesterol, a healthy weight, abstaining from smoking, or exercising regularly (Levy et al., 2002).

Performance Piece: Woman as Spectacle

The first appearance of the "chorus of resonant voices" that I will introduce throughout this paper is my own, in a very particular context. This is a small portion of a performance piece. *Woman as Spectacle*:

At my age (chronological, that is), I am meant to disappear. I should have
been gone long ago. In the dance of the life cycle, I am being propelled
against the wall. Centrifugal forces spin me to the chairs from which I
rose so long ago . . . arms that circled me and kept me on the floor. Oh,
how I could dance . . . . Now they've let me go. My dance card is empty.
Now I'm melding with the walls, pressing into the paper, melting into the
glue, stuck, not pinned and wiggling, like Eliot's Prufrock, but misting
into mottled lavender, without a muscle's twitch. This is the fate of a
woman of a mature age. She is somewhere over 40, and, according to
some, about as useful as a fruit fly (at least they have the courtesy to
die swiftly when their breeding days are done). If she cannot procreate,
she is lifeless, you see, but not dead. She never should attract our gaze;
she learns to be the anti-spectacle . . . .

Such hatred we sometimes feel for her. That shameful blot on the
image of our youth. Couldn't we just wring her neck? Be done with
her. No one needs her. Hoarder of Medicare. Social Security sad sack.
Our tax dollars feeding a body no one wants to see.

But lest we discard her so quickly. She is me, and perhaps you. She is
our destiny. (M. Gergen, 2001, pp. 176–177)

The Social Reconstruction of Aging

Stereotypes are important because they have consequences for how we
interact with one another. Although they are often very powerful cultural
constructions that are built and maintained through public and private use,
they can be changed. The basic philosophical stance that supports this position is social constructionism (Gergen, 2009; Gergen & Gergen, 2004;
Greene, 2003). Social constructions posits that the "realities" of the world
are created and stabilized by social groups that support their essences for
a variety of reasons. Conceptions of aging and of the human being more generally, are created through the culture's constructions of them. But so too are
other features of society, such as the division of people into two genders,
three sexual orientations (or could it be four?), five social classes, and other
"realities" such as "death," "taxes," and "rocks," not to mention "rock 'n'
roll." This is not to say that social constructionists are solipsists, who believe
that nothing exists at all, but rather that whatever there is comes into being
for us as we develop meaning through our communicative processes. The
positive side of this perspective is that even though the negative stereotypes
of aging are powerful, there are possibilities for changing them.

CHANGING STEREOTYPES AND PROMOTING
ALTERNATIVE VISIONS

Much of my work in psychology has been devoted to this aim and to helping
promote alternatives visions. This work has taken various forms, including

joining with Ken Gergen in editing the *Positive Aging Newsletter*, a bimonthly electronic newsletter that publishes research and newsworthy items that contradict the negative stereotypes and support positive potentials for aging. This electronic newsletter has grown over the years to almost 20,000 subscribers and is now translated into several languages. This project has exposed me to various professional publications devoted to aging; I have learned much about the tendency in every gerontological field—social work, psychology, nursing, and sociology, among others—to emphasize the negative. The typical journal on aging has a vast majority of articles on decline and decrepitude. It is no wonder that professionals and the public alike believe that aging is a scary and depressing eventuality.

At the same time, in our search for the positive possibilities, I have become much more optimistic and enthusiastic about the potentials of aging. Our newsletter proposes that aging can be a stage of "unprecedented human development." We reject the common stereotypes and the developmental literature that suggests that the aging process is an arc, with our youthful years spent in reaching the apex and our mature years in sliding down the other side. This metaphor of the arc always leads us to a long and dismal end. The approach we take in the newsletter does just the opposite; we emphasize the multiple potentials for people as they age. Along with certain other gerontologists, we suggest the possibility of an endless upward spiral, with multiple trajectories (Diener et al., 1999). We recognize that just as adolescents are quite diverse, despite their common age range, there is also diversity among older people. For some, pleasure is taken in the "sybaritic lifestyle" of leisure and relaxation (Gergen & Gergen, 2000); for some, pleasure is in new work, new careers, and new challenges (Baltes & Baltes, 1990); for others, a new identity as an artist is acquired through discipline and training in the postcareer years (Cohen, 2006); and for some, a life is founded on service to others, in the manner of Jimmy and Roselyn Carter, who have found great rewards in solving world problems, and also of Bill and Melinda Gates, with their foundation's international work.

Conversation on a Tennis Court

A second appearance of the "chorus of resonant voices" provides a lived example of this redefinition of aging. It took place between players on a tennis court recently. I overheard the following exchange:

> JAN: I may not be able to play tennis too often in the fall. I'm going to be going to a studio in Haverford.
> ANN: What are you going to be doing there?
> JAN: I'm going to an art class. Going to draw nude bodies." (*She laughs a bit nervously.*) It's something that I've been wanting to do for a long time.

ANN: I didn't know you were an artist.

JAN: Oh, I would never call myself that. It is just something I've always wanted to do, and finally, now that I've retired, I am going to do something I was never permitted to do.

ANN: What did you do before you retired?

JAN: I was a hospital administrator. It wasn't very exciting. Being an artist has always been my dream, and now finally I am going to be permitted to do it.

As I listened, I wondered who was doing the permitting. Was it she herself that was finally giving herself permission? This conversation seemed to suggest the beginning formation of the butterfly from the chrysalis stage.

The Power of Numbers: Baby Boomers and Beyond

There are means of moving toward a positive reconstruction of aging. I consider here two major contributions: the contribution of the current historical moment and the positive resources available in daily relations.

For many decades, beginning with the first wave of postwar babies, the "baby boomers" have had a felt presence in society. This generation has the numbers to greatly alter how the "third age" of life might be construed. Today, instead of being a small minority in the general population, people over 50 have become a dominant group. By 2030, one in five Americans will be 65 or older, and the majority of them will be women (Hagestad, 1991). When there are many people in a social category, they have the opportunity to change the nature of society. They can generate resistance to undesirable things and create a mutually supported vision of other preferred alternatives, especially if they have been used to expressing their views over the life course.

One way older people can have an impact on society is through the political process. The percentage of older people who vote far exceeds that of those in their 20s. According to the U.S. Bureau of the Census, 72% of Americans 65 to 74 voted in the 2000 national elections, compared with 33% of those 18 to 24. In Iowa, for example, 84% of the eligible voters in the 65 to 74 bracket voted in 2000, compared to the state average of 64%. In the last general election in 2006, almost 52% of those who cast a ballot were 50 years old or older.

Because of this ballot box power, politicians take older people very seriously. In fact, Tip O'Neill, former U.S. Congressman from Massachusetts, once described programs such as Social Security and Medicare as the "third rail" of American politics, "touch it and you die" (Morris, 1996, p. xi). Discussions of social security can be viewed as dangerous for any political party that might want to curtail payments, reduce benefits, or invite risk, regardless of the "health" of the fund.

Generally, baby boomers and those who are older are also surprisingly well-to-do. As a group, those over 65 control 70% of the total national wealth (Dychwald, 1999). Once upon a time, the poorest people in the country were the elderly. Today, the average 70-year-old is richer than the average 30 year old, although certainly not all older people share alike in this bounty. Over time this power is becoming recognizable in the marketplace and the media. While the most prominent images of women continue to be young, slim, and sexy, there are some signs that the advertising industry is beginning to create messages and images that are attracting older consumers. The Dove Soap campaign, which featured women who were not professional models, was a pioneer; other companies that are heeding the demographic shifts, especially cosmetic, clothing, pharmaceuticals, perfume, and travel-oriented enterprises, are using older people.

RELATIONAL RESOURCES FOR POSITIVE AGING

Wealth is More Than Money

While the relative wealth of those over 60 can be documented, researchers have also found other forms of security in parts of the older population. The "chorus of resonant elders" must include African-American women and their contribution to our alternative vision of aging. Here is a summary of a report on their perspective: Money isn't everything. This is the attitude of many poor minority group women who were studied by gerontologists interested in what helps poor women cope. Despite low incomes and financial problems at home, older African-American women who have strong church ties are relatively happy. (Elderly, single African-American women fare among the worst economically in the U. S. today. In general, older widows are twice as likely to be below the poverty line than single men.) They are confident that they have a place to go for comfort, for friendship, and sometimes for various forms of material support. It is also a place where members of the congregation can enact the civic responsibility that historically the church has upheld (Carlton-LaNey, 2007). Among older African Americans, religious involvement is associated with physical health and psychological well-being. Being religious is more important to health status than financial well-being (Larson, Sherrill, & Lyons, 1999).

It is through social interchange that meaning is constructed. Thus, the most important means of replacing the myths of old age with more positive outlook is to gather relational forces that together can engage in transformation. Existing research lends strong support to this view. Having close friends, partners, children, and others who care about you and whom you care about are among the most crucial contributors to a satisfying life. An often-unrecognized source of social interchange and connection is with people in the workplace as well as with others in public settings where one might do volunteer work or engage in consumer activities.

In a study of German elders, researchers concluded that age was not a central factor in how satisfied or emotionally rich one's life is. Even physical decline was not a powerful predictor of life satisfaction. The researchers suggested that many physical changes are seen "as trivial... a normal part of the aging process" (p. 371). Among the most important contributors to satisfaction were one's companions, especially close friends. They proved more important than family connections or financial wealth (Steverink et al., 2001).

Traditionally it has been found that being married is a strong correlate of a healthy and happy old age, but what is at the core of this correlation is the intimate connections that people who are married often have (Argyle, 1999; Myers, 1993). If there are close friends, children, or neighbors with whom one has open and caring relationships, marriage is not essential for a happy life. For men, marriage has been more significant than for women in this regard, but this is because men are less likely to have and keep close friends in their mature years (Gannon, 1999). Research on relations with children suggest that the "empty nest" syndrome—that people are miserable when the last child leaves home—is a myth. The most difficult time of life for parents is when the children are at home, and life improves considerably when they leave (Neugarten, 1979). At the same time, parents who continue to assist their children with material assets are less likely to be depressed than those who don't, and they are especially pleased if their children acknowledge their beneficence (Byers, Levy, & Allore, 2008). The "chorus of resonant voices" might chime in here with a saying: "The only symptom of the empty nest syndrome that has been found is a smile."

In 2002, the Chicago Health, Aging, and Social Relations Study examined the relationships of social life to well-being (Cacioppo et al., 2002). The study began with 230 English-speaking Chicagoans between the ages of 50 and 67 from the African-American, Hispanic, and Caucasian populations. Previous studies had shown that socially engaged people were more likely to have lower blood pressure and better sleep quality than more isolated people. Although there were no differences between solitary and sociable people in terms of hours of sleep, those who slept alone had a poorer quality of sleep, and their bodies did not have the same opportunities to restore themselves as more sociable sleepers had. Neighborhood life also made a difference in people's self-rated health scores. The impact of neighborhood was dependent on how people felt about it. If someone felt comfortable and integrated into the area, that person tended to feel more robust, regardless of how poor the area was in economic terms. If there is one message from these data, it is that people need people, as the song goes.

Although cultural stereotypes suggest that older people are not interested in romance and sexuality, research indicates this is not the case. Having a romantic partner is strongly related to feelings of satisfaction in life.

A survey conducted by the National Council on Aging indicated that 70% of sexually active women over 60 reported being as satisfied or more satisfied with their sexual lives now as when they were in their 40s (Price, 2006). In a study of over 400 older women in the United States, approximately 40% said that their sexual desire was the same or greater than it had ever been (Kliger & Nedelman, 2006). Often the increased sexuality was related to their increased appreciation for other sensual sources, such as perfumes, flowers, soft fabrics, music, and massage. The proliferation of spas in the United States would attest to this yearning for sensual touch. Over the life course, many women who have had heterosexual relations, including years of marriage and children, choose a woman as an intimate partner (Gabbay & Wahler, 2002; Hall & Fine, 2005). Little research has been reported about lesbians in later life, but the available data suggest that, contrary to the stereotype that older lesbians are lonely and bereft of close personal relationships, they are more likely to be deeply involved in gratifying relationships that include affection and support. Interviews with 20 lesbian women aged 50 to 73 indicate that they have developed strong friendship networks that often supplant familial ties, which may be weak or missing. For many women, the option of choosing a woman to love was restricted by cultural, familial, and religious norms, and only in later life did this lifestyle become possible (Goldman, 2006b; Jensen, 1999). Another "resonant voice," speaking for a changed view of older women, is a woman who entered a lesbian relationship for the first time, in later life. She says:

> Sharing my life with Grace has made me a healthier, stronger, and better person. This second half of our lives is, as the psychologist Carl Jung said, a moving toward fullness of being. Grace helps me do this. I can trust my heart and soul and body to her, and that's extremely important and comforting. (Goldman, 2006a)

Extending the Reach of Important Relationships

Nor is it essential that one's participation in relationships be confined to the near and dear. Interest groups, clubs, organizations, political parties, may all stimulate interest, enthusiasm, and active engagement in the world. One shining example, having fun and being outrageous, is The Red Hat Society, an international organization dedicated to repelling the stereotypes of aging women (Cooper, 2004). The group takes its emblematic red hat from the poem, "Warning" by Jenny Joseph, which begins, "When I am an old woman I shall wear purple, with a red hat which doesn't go, and doesn't suit me."

Many women become involved in the arts and other intellectual and cultural pursuits. They may take up drawing and painting, sculpture, pottery, music lessons, join a theater group, take academic courses, or volunteer for civic and cultural activities. Gene Cohen (2000, 2006) has written about the powers of the aging brain and the potential for the development of artistic vocations among older people. Cohen stresses that this is not only a time for dilettante pleasures, dabbling in the arts, but also a time for serious, professional level engagement in music, art, or literature. Through discipline and dedication, older artists and musicians can compete with younger colleagues. The notion that only young people can acquire the skills for high-level artistic performance is another anti-aging myth.

Aging has been associated with retirement, both from work and from the world more generally. Early gerontologists made the claim that disengagement was the appropriate theme for older people (Cummings & Henry, 1961). Today, the theoretical position in gerontology that is most accepted advocates activity and involvement for older people (Hazan, 1994). This position holds that having activities that engage one, of any sort, is preferable to distancing oneself from ongoing activities.

The meaning of retirement has changed greatly in the past 50 years, partially due to the fact that the average life expectancy has grown. A retired worker at 65 today may anticipate at least 10 more years of life, if not 20 or 30, after traditional employment ceases. Retirement may indicate a cessation of one's primary employment commitment(s), but it is not the end of productive engagement in the world. The "New Retirement" baby boomers demonstrate how postcareer life may be lived. A Pew Foundation report indicates that 71% of current workers think they will continue to work after retirement, more from desire than necessity. A 2005 study by Merrill Lynch found that 76% of baby boomers expect to retire around age 64 and then start entirely new jobs or careers (Wright, 2006).

Many older people find significant social engagement in volunteer work. Some work with children and youth as tutors, Big Brothers or Big Sisters, or by serving in advisory capacities for youth related programs. In Florida, for example, children from families below the poverty line who maintain good grades and school attendance receive special attention weekly from an older person who helps to guide them and support them in their academic work. The rewards for the students include college tuition scholarships at state schools, and the rewards for both student and adult-friend are multiple. In a variety of programs across the country, older adults are serving as role models for the young, and they, at the same time, are benefiting from being brought into the worlds of these children (Windsor, Anstey, & Rogers, 2008).

Caring Relationships from Cross-Generational Volunteer Work

Another of the "resonant voices" speaking for the ways that older women are changing the meaning of aging is that of Sylvia, a volunteer in a cross-generational outreach program. I summarize her experience here:

Sylvia, was assigned to help Cristina, a fourth grade girl from an immigrant family who was unable to read English. Sylvia, who was 65, had problems walking; she had arthritis and used a cane. Twice a week Sylvia and Cristina met in the cafeteria and then walked to the library, which was on the second floor of an adjacent building. At first, it was quite a struggle for Sylvia to make the walk, and for Cristina, it was slow going with the reading. At the end of each session, they would walk together to the gates of the school to say good-bye. During the course of the semester, Sylvia, who had not previously been exercising, began to have more mobility and less pain in her legs, and by the end of the semester, no longer needed her cane. Cristina finally caught on to reading and had reached grade level, much to the joy of her teachers, Sylvia, and herself.

THERAPY AS SOCIAL TRANSFORMATION

My hope has been to offer resources that might assist therapists who are working with the aging population to move toward a transformation in their awareness of concepts about age and in their recognition of the potentials of aging. At present there is not enough work being done to support therapists in this vital area of inquiry. In a search for literature to inform their therapeutic work, Fredman, Anderson, and Stott (in press) found

> no books that specifically addressed therapeutic practice with older people, in the contexts of power and discrimination, in relation to gender, race, sexuality, physical and cognitive ability and, of course, age. We also did not find any publications specifically offering guiding principles for working therapeutically with older people in the contexts of the complex webs of medical and social services that are often involved with their care. (in press)

Because of its relative position of authority in society, the therapeutic community can make a significant contribution to the process of transformation in the field of gerontology while simultaneously serving as a major resource for clients. At the outset, this mission may entail challenging the negative stereotypes so common to the culture. For example, it may mean challenging older clients who have themselves incorporated the negative stereotypes and who might believe, for example, that they are too old to take up new ventures or to start a new relationship because there is no future in it. The greatest danger of therapy would be to have therapists supporting the passive, disengagement model of aging. Another theme that therapists might well support is that the healthy human being is a social being who thrives on being deeply engaged with others. Instead of promoting the old cultural myth that the healthy individual is an independent, autonomous one, therapists might help to influence clients in finding richer and more diverse social networks to support their growth. It is also important for therapists to search their own hearts as they engage in work with older people.

Therapists Join the Chorus of Voices who Resonate with a New Vision of Aging

Not surprisingly, psychotherapists number among the "chorus of resonant voices" who are challenging their own ageism and helping their clients, and their culture, to do the same. Psychotherapists Fredman and colleagues (in press) work in a highly personal and collaborative way. In the early stages of their efforts, they realized that their own histories with older people and that their feelings and opinions about aging could affect—for good or ill—their therapeutic practices. Thus, they met together to tell memory stories. They found themselves deeply moved by their stories, and they began to reflect on the themes emerging from them. These deliberations were then linked to more general theoretical formulations in systemic therapy. The results were salutary. As they put it, "Our telling, re-telling and reflecting on the tellings of our memories enabled us to become observers of our selves and of our discourses and thus we were able to question the ethics of our practice. In this way we were enabled to find ways of looking that oriented our future practice so that we found new ways to go on" (Gergen & Gergen, in press b).

It is important for therapists to recognize that, regardless of age, people desire many of the same things. Working in favor of positive therapeutic outcomes is that, in general, older people have an advantage over younger people in emotional stability and complexity. Older people tend to be less emotionally labile than younger people when it comes to matters of love and loss, health and illness, good times and bad (Lockenhoff, Costa, & Lane, 2008). They are better at coping with adversity and in handling disappointments. One might say older people are more resilient to the stresses of life (Gergen & Gergen, in press a). They are also better able to take a philosophical perspective on issues, and, thus, are often said to possess wisdom, a trait reserved for the old (Baltes & Staudinger, 2000). These psychological tendencies are resources that can aid the therapist in working with a client.

The therapist can also serve as a supportive guide during the inevitable transitional challenges of aging, such as painful separations, illnesses, and other losses. The hope would be that therapists could open the door to a more enriched form of life for the aging, regardless of the difficulties that may beset them.

Ideally, we should move beyond the medical metaphor in working with many of the problems encountered by the elderly. Much of the distress and anguish of aging is culturally produced. These are problems in part because of the cultural stereotypes of what constitutes worth, the nature of love, good looks, and the fully functioning body. I am proposing that it is not the therapist's task to solve the problems in the terms supplied by the culture but by helping clients to generate a new vision of aging. Therapists can share a therapeutic vision that helps their clients realize the positive potential of aging. It is the possibility of living within this new vision of a richer and more engaged form of life that can be realized. In these ways, therapists, as societal change agents, help bring new life to old bodies.

Voices Throughout the Planet, Across the Generations

The Taos Institute, a think-tank on aging, recently held a conference in Sarasota, Florida. (To see the archives of the *Positive Aging Newsletter* go to TaosInsitute.net.) Among the attendees were three psychology graduate students from Roskilde University in Denmark. They asked to interview Ken Gergen and me on positive aging as part of their dissertation work. Mille, an outgoing and enthusiastic 24-year-old with the typical Scandinavian blond hair and eyes as blue as a Siamese cat was impressed with the conference and the older people who had presented there. At the conclusion of our interview, she burst out, "Oh, I want to be old! I want to have gray hair now and be so wise and enjoy life so much as all the people here. I can hardly wait to be old, like you all are."

REFERENCES

Argyle, M. (1999). Causes and correlates of happiness. In D. Kahneman, E. Diener, & N. Schwartz (Eds.), *Foundations of hedonic psychology: Scientific perspectives on enjoyment and suffering* (pp. 651–652). New York: Russell Sage.

Baltes, P. B., & Baltes, M. M. (Eds.). (1990). *Successful aging.* New York: Cambridge University Press.

Baltes, P. B., & Staudinger, U. M. (2000). Wisdom: A metaheuristic (pragmatic) to orchestrate mind and virtue toward excellence. *American Psychologist, 55,* 122–136.

Byers, A. L., Levy, B. R., & Allore, H. G. (2008). When parents matter to their adult children: Filial reliance associated with parents' depressive symptoms. *Journal of Gerontology, 63,* 33–40.

Cacioppo, J. T., Hawkley, L. C., Rickett, E. M., & Masi, C. M. (2002). Sociality, spirituality, and meaning making: Chicago health, aging and social relations study. *Review of General Psychology, 9,* 143–155.

Carlton-LaNey, I. (2007). "Doing the lord's work": Civic engagement. *Generations, 30,* 47–50.

Cohen, G. (2000). *The creative age: Awakening human potential in the second half of life.* New York: Harper Collins/Avon books.

Cohen G. (2006). *The mature mind: The positive power of the aging brain.* New York: Basic Books.

Cooper, S. E. (2004). *The Red Hat Society: Fun and friendship after 50.* New York: Time Warner Books.

Cummings, E., & Henry, H. (1961). *Growing old.* New York: Basic Books.

Daniluk, J. (1998). *Women's sexuality across the life span: Challenging myths, creating meaning.* New York: Guilford.

Diener, E., Suh, E. M., Lucas, R. E., & Smith, H. L. (1999). Subjective well-being: Three decades of progress. *Psychological Bulletin, 125,* 276–302.

Dychwald, K. (1999). *Age power: How the 21st century will be ruled by the new old.* New York: Penguin.

Fredman, G., Anderson, E., & Stott, J. (Eds.) (in press). *Being with older people: A systemic approach.* London: Karnac Books.

Freud, S. (1927). Some psychological consequences of the anatomic distinction between the sexes. *Journal of Psycho-Analysis, 8,* 133–142.

Gabbay, S. F., & Wahler, J. J. (2002). Lesbian aging: Review of a growing literature. *Journal of Gay and Lesbian Social Services, 14,* 1–21.

Gannon, L. R. (1999). *Women and aging.* New York: Routledge.

Gergen, K. J. (2009). *Invitations to social constructionism* (2nd ed.). London: Sage.

Gergen, K. J., & Gergen, M. (2000). The new aging: Self construction and social values. In K. W. Schaie (Ed.), *Social structures and aging* (pp. 281–306). New York: Springer.

Gergen, K. J., & Gergen, M. (2004). *Social construction: Entering the dialogue.* Chagrin Falls, OH: Taos Institute Publications.

Gergen, K. J., & Gergen, M. (In press a). Positive aging: Resilience and reconstruction. In P. S. Fry & C. L. M. Keyes (Eds.), *Frontiers of resilient aging.* Cambridge, UK: Cambridge University Press.

Gergen, K. J., & Gergen, M. (In press b). Working with elders: Inspiring the young. In G. Fredman, E. Anderson, & J. Stott (Eds.), *Being with older people: A systemic approach.* London: Karnac Books.

Gergen, M. (1990). Finished at forty: Women's development within the patriarchy. *Psychology of Women Quarterly, 14,* 451–470.

Gergen, M. (2001). *Feminist reconstructions in psychology: Narrative, gender and performance.* Thousand Oaks, CA: Sage.

Goldman, C. (2006a, August 18). Late-life love: The final (blog) chapter. Retrieved October 16, 2008, from http://www.thirdage.com/today/aging-well/late-life-love-the-final-blog-chapter.

Goldman, C. (2006b). *Late-life love: Romance and new relationships in later years.* Chagrin Falls, OH: Fairview Press.

Greene, S. (2003). *The psychological development of girls and women: Rethinking change in time.* New York: Routledge.

Hagestad, G. O. (1991). The aging society as a context for family life. In N. A. S. Jecker (Ed.), *Aging and ethics: Philosophical problems in gerontology. Contemporary issues in biomedicine, ethics, and society* (pp. 123–146). Clifton, NJ: Humana Press.

Hall, R. L., & Fine, M. (2005). The stories we tell: The lives and friendship of two older black lesbians. *Psychology of Women Quarterly, 29,* 177–187.

Hazan, H. (1994). *Old age: Constructions and deconstructions.* Cambridge: Cambridge University Press.

Jensen, K. (1999). *Lesbian epiphanies: Women coming out in later life.* Binghamton, NY: Haworth Press.

Kliger, L., & Nedelman, D. (2006). *Still sexy after all these years? The nine unspoken truths about women's desire.* New York: Penguin/Perigee.

Larson, D. B., Sherrill, K. A., & Lyons, S. S. (1999). What do we really know about religion and health among the aging populations? In J. S. Levin (Ed.), *Religion in aging and health* (pp. 183–199). London: Sage.

Levy, B. R., Slade, M. D., Kunkel, S. R., & Kasl, S. V. (2002). Longevity increased by positive self-perceptions of aging. *Journal of Personality and Social Psychology, 83,* 261–270.

Lockenhoff, C. E., Costa, Jr. P. T., & Lane, R. D. (2008). Age differences in descriptions of emotional experiences in oneself and others. *Journal of Gerontology, 63,* 192–199.

Martin, E. (1999). Medical metaphors of women's bodies: Menstruation and menopause. In K. Charmaz & D. Paterniti (Eds.), *Health, illness, and healing: Society, social context, and self* (pp. 292–293). Los Angeles: Roxbury.

Morris, C. R. (1996). *The AARP: American's most powerful lobby and the clash of generations.* New York: Random House.

Myers, D. G. (1993). *The pursuit of happiness.* New York: Avon.

Nelson, T. D. (Ed.) (2002). *Ageism: Stereotyping and prejudice against older persons.* Cambridge, MA: MIT Press.

Neugarten, B. L. (1979). Time, age, and the life cycle. *American Journal of Psychiatry, 136,* 887–894.

Price, J. (2006). *Better than I ever expected: Straight talk about sex after sixty.* New York: Seal Press.

Schmidt, P. J., & Rubinow, D. R. (1991). Menopause-related affective disorders: A justification for further study. *American Journal of Psychiatry, 148,* 844–852.

Shih, M., Pittinsky, T. L., & Ambady, N. (1999). Stereotype susceptibility: Identity salience and shifts in quantitative performance. *Psychological Science, 10,* 880–883.

Steele, C. M. (1997). A threat in the air: How stereotypes shape intellectual identity and performance. *American Psychologist, 52,* 613–629.

Steverink, N., Westerhof, G. J., Bode, C., & Dittmann-Kohli, F. (2001). The personal experience of aging, individual resources, and subjective well-being. *Journal of Gerontology, 56,* 364–373.

Windsor, R. D., Anstey, K. J., & Rodgers, B. T. (2008). Volunteering and psychological well-being among young-old adults: How much is too much? *The Gerontologist, 48,* 59–70.

Wright, C. L. (2006, November 15). Changing directions and finding yourself. *New York Times,* 7.

Reflections on Aging, Psychotherapy, and Spiritual Practice

ARLENE BERMANN

Private Practice, San Francisco and Marin, California

This article, written by a therapist in midlife, considers the intersection of aging, psychotherapy, and spiritual practice. It includes professional and personal reflections as well as clinical examples explored through the complementary lenses of intersubjectivity theory, which describes the co-creation of experience by therapist and patient, and Zen Buddhsim, which explores the illusory nature of some of our most basic assumptions. The author discusses the nuances of listening to and attempting to understand others, especially in the transference and countertransference. The author reflects on her personal experience of the processes of aging and maturing, both emotionally and physically, and on ways in which life has changed for her, over time, as a result of aging, meditation, and psychotherapy practice. Concepts explored include co-creation of relationship, emptiness and impermanence, and existential anxiety.

Having turned 50 recently, I'm feeling lucky to be alive. And having practiced psychotherapy, on both sides of the couch, as well as Zen Buddhist meditation, for much of my life, I can now appreciate the extent to which these practices have ripened through the years, softening me up, helping me to loosen my grip. They've been working on me as I've aged, deepening and widening my understanding of life's possibilities. When I speak of life's possibilities, I refer to those times when the wall we think is *just-the-way-life-is* dissolves, shifting our horizon and expanding the space within which we live.

THE BENEFITS OF AGING AND PRACTICING TO MY WORK: A CLINICAL EXAMPLE

A few years ago, after the December holidays, my patient Roxanne came for a session and asked me about how my vacation had been. I've always felt awkward in response to this question. It's a question that, for me, points out the ways in which the therapeutic relationship is asymmetrical, and in which I am unknown to my patients. I feel the echo of this in the patient's question, and sometimes it evokes a longing, which the patient may share, for a different kind of connection. Sometimes the question provokes the opposite: a desire in me for distance, for protection from this question and the many feelings for which it is a messenger. Then I might feel some guilt toward the patient for my own emotional response. Either way, when this question arises it puts me in touch with some of the sadness I feel at the limitations of the therapeutic relationship. And if anything, this sadness and discomfort has increased as I've aged, not decreased.

Furthermore, embedded in this moment is my tendency to feel ashamed about my awkwardness, as if I should be really relaxed about this, I should welcome this opportunity for a slightly different way of relating. Instead I have tended to judge myself as uptight, a "withholding therapist," a therapist who shouldn't feel this way. Although over the years I have sometimes answered the question comfortably, it is more usual for me to feel some uncertainty.

On the day when Roxanne asked I was acutely aware of the fact that I had had a terrible vacation, and this left me in a bind. I want to be truthful with my patients, and it seemed hard to disclose just a little of this negativity without burdening Roxanne and eliciting sympathetic further inquiry. When Roxanne asked about my vacation, my tension level shot up, and I deflected the question. I avoided eye contact and said that my vacation was fine in a perfunctory way, and then I quickly smiled. My smile, I'm sure, was like a door slamming shut, and my whole response was unconscious code for "let's move on, I'm not going to be with you here." Not only did I try to avoid Roxanne, but I lied. Well, not exactly. More to the point, I felt like I was lying.

Roxanne smiled angrily back at me and I thought I saw her roll her eyes a little. Luckily, we had the benefit of years of treatment and of some success with difficult interpersonal work between us, and so I was able to override my impulse to ignore her nonverbal protest and I invited her into a conversation about our situation. I knew my inquiry might feel dangerous or blaming to her, but being less timid about these things than I'd have been years before, I persisted anyway. And Roxanne had enough confidence to give voice to her reactions. She said accusingly that my response made her feel like she was prying, that I was saying she needed to carry all the weight of our conversation all the time, and that she was unwelcome. She felt that I was holding a boundary in a way that felt excluding, and it felt especially painful after being disconnected during my vacation.

I felt caught, and yet I was glad to be caught by Roxanne. When I was younger, I was rarely glad to be caught by a patient; in fact, it never seemed like quite the right time. Now I had more facility with the experience. I might say that as a result of age, and my practices, I was a bit more able to relax into my discomfort than I had been in the past. As I contained my anxiety, Roxanne and I were able to name what didn't happen: the way I didn't truly receive the question, meet her gaze, or answer authentically. I simply hadn't known how to answer her, hadn't had access to any response that had felt deeply right. I had done my best, and it had felt hurtful to Roxanne. Roxanne and I then noticed together how attuned she is to my tension level, to any rebuff, and to the experience of being left alone to carry the weight of relationship, all of which were traumatic themes in her childhood. We were able to look at how the question represented a longing for more contact and how, at the same time, it was a likely setup for a disappointment and a painful exchange. Once Roxanne felt understood by me, she was able to talk about her feeling that her mother withheld herself sadistically, rejecting Roxanne's attempts to know what was in her mother's mind and heart. I had the opportunity then to connect with Roxanne about these painful memories in a live way, based on the transaction we'd just lived through together.

After much discussion, I was able to share that I hadn't meant to reject her, and to disclose aspects of my experience of the difficulty between us, including my dilemma regarding the less than happy vacation. Levenson (in Bromberg, 1998) writes, "Catching the therapist in a self-serving operation may do more for the patient's sense of competence than a lifetime of benevolent participations" (p. 282). And so it seemed to be, as my disclosure brought visible relief to Roxanne. Roxanne and I had a trying history together, and it had often been difficult to discuss our relationship without us both having a powerful sense of imminent danger. This discussion enabled us to become closer, more attuned with each other, a critical thing in the course of a difficult therapy.

Had this happened 10 years ago, the outcome would have been different. Ten years ago my tension would have been even higher, and the patient, sensing this, would likely have protected me more from her reaction to me, just as she did with her fragile and highly narcissistic parents. Also, it would have taken me longer to come clean, and I would have been less open to a full exploration of her experience because I was less comfortable with my own blunders 10 years ago than I am now. Years ago, I was less able to tolerate angry accusation, or else tolerate blame and accusation. And if we hadn't fully permitted Roxanne's accusations and explored her experience it wouldn't have been possible for me to make the self-disclosures that I made. Years ago, we likely wouldn't have slowed down, taken our time, and looked together as closely and honestly at the moment we were co-creating, or at the moment that was creating us. Years ago, we might not have gotten to see how perfect the difficulties between us were or what opportunities for healing they contained.

EMPTINESS, IMPERMANENCE, AND PERCEPTION

A young intern once came to me with concern that her patient was, as she said, "going on and on about his problems ad nauseum." When I asked how long she'd been seeing him, she said for four weeks. I encouraged this intern to approach her patient as if she had endless time and patience with which to be curious and to learn about him. When she returned for her next supervision, she told me that this had become one of her most interesting clinical relationships. This reminded me of my own past experience. Years ago, when patients gave very subtle nonverbal cues that their subject matter was unimportant, I believed them and became anxious with them about whether we were wasting time. Together then, we tended to close down the therapeutic space. As I matured, I could see beyond the surface and take the cue that the patient required extra permission to elaborate her narrative, and we could discover the riches below this tendency to contract.

These examples, in which the patient feels unimportant or undeserving and the therapist begins to join the patient in her inhibition, can each be described as psychoanalytic, intersubjective phenomena that are instructive about both the patient's and the clinician's object relational worlds. We can hypothesize that my intern's patient was dismissed or invisible in some way in his family, or alternately that he felt overly scrutinized and so receded in interpersonal situations. In response, the therapist might feel ineffective (especially if she is an intern), or helpless, and her strategies for coping with these feelings will also have their own genetic origins.

This situation can also be viewed through the lens of Buddhist psychology, which opens a window onto transcendent understandings regarding the insubstantiality or emptiness of phenomenon and its impermanence. One way to think about this is to consider that each moment in time represents a birth and death of our world, and that each moment is then strung together with the next by our minds, forming a perception that things are solid and time is linear. We might consider our bodies as a concrete image of this— our bodies—which appear to be solid and fixed. On closer examination though, our cells are being born and dying all the time, and in this way we ourselves are experiencing birth and death continuously. Thich Nhat Hanh, addressing these issues, helps us see how human perception is organized in ways that make it hard to see clearly:

> ... it is very easy to confuse our mental image, our sign of something, with its reality. The process of mistaking our perceptions for reality is so subtle that it is very difficult to know what is going on, but we must try not to do

this. The way to avoid this is mindfulness. We practice meditation to train the mind in direct perception . . . the person we love is not a real person, but an image created by our consciousness. This false perception can create suffering. Sitting in the car next to our spouse, we completely ignore her because we think that we already know everything about her and that there is nothing interesting to learn about her anymore . . . scientists have acknowledged that they don't even know what a speck of dust is. Looking deeply into an electron, we bow our heads in awe. And yet here is a human being sitting next to us and we think we already know everything about her. We hate or love depending on images we ourselves create . . . . Our consciousness rarely touches reality. (Hahn, 2001, pp. 25, 50, 51)

The commitment to looking and listening more deeply, to trying to see and hear the person before us, requires that we hold our perceptions lightly and that we let go of our ideas as the ever-changing realities of clinical relationships present themselves. The constraining notions of self and other that we create in each therapeutic relationship must be born and die, repeatedly, if our clinical work is to have life in it. Studying emptiness and insubstantiality, in psychotherapy and in life, can bring joy but also invites mourning. Donnell Stern (2003) gives a feeling for the sadness that this entails in clinical work, particularly for clinicians who have practiced over time, in his book *Unformulated Experience*:

> Since each understanding is contextual, what Issacharoff and Hunt (1978) call a "new truth," it will be displaced by fresh understanding as the work proceeds. There is an excitement to this, but also a kind of sadness, because every new truth becomes a prejudice. Every understanding is eventually a betrayal. Analysts are always on the verge of relinquishing their proudest moments, understandings that sometimes have been hoped for and awaited over long periods of time. (p. 252)

ILLUSIONS AND WHAT LIFE IS

I've been having a cure fantasy and dyeing my hair for some years now, despite evidence that it is bad for my health. This is a rejection of my own aging and a fierce form of clinging: to the rich brownness of my youthful hair, to my love of youth, to my wish to avoid my vulnerabilities. I've been avoiding my own reactions to my aging each day as I look in the mirror, and also avoiding the negative judgments of aging women in our culture as I navigate the world. I will appear differently with gray hair, and I used to hope that when I did let it gray, it would give me the appearance of a youthful, prematurely gray woman. I've mused wishfully about the beautiful white hair some women have, the kind that looks brilliant, like an alternative form of youthfulness, the kind that seems to defy the brittleness, diminishments, and grayness that can come with age.

By dyeing my hair, I've been dodging one of death's signals, and missing out on an opportunity to mourn the irretrievable loss of my younger self. I've also been a participant in a strange cultural illusion: if women en masse stopped dyeing their hair, our visual cultural landscape would actually be quite different than it is now. It might be a relief to all of us if that happened, once we'd all adjusted.

We invoke these fantasies of cure to cope with our anxieties—our anxieties about ourselves, our loneliness, our desires, our physical pain, our deaths. Fantasies of cure, whether pursued through hair dye, work achievements, romance, remodeling, psychotherapy, or spiritual practice do seem to break down as we age and as we practice, if we're lucky. Now, we hope to help our patients expand their notions of what is possible in life, to ask for more of what they truly desire, at the same time we hope to help them to let go of illusions of cure. It helps if, as we therapists age and as we practice, we manage to become dis-illusioned ourselves, so that we may enter more deeply into the body of our own lives. Everything we do in this regard communicates itself to our patients.

It is in midlife that "one first deals with loss of youth, tries to match the percept of an aging self with the mental image of a younger self, begins to perceive the passage of time differently, and personalizes death with an accompanying realization of a finite amount of time left to live" (Ellman, 1996, pp. 354–355). But that disjunction between the mental image of our youthful selves and the person in the mirror is hard to accept, especially for women. I encountered forceful resistance at the hair salon when I once announced that I was considering letting my hair go gray. The strength of the response shocked me. The simple mention of this possibility elicited a storm of rejection: "No!" the women cried, in a chorus, "You're too young for that!" But I wasn't too young. I was 46 at the time, and as far as I can tell there's no arguing with my hair, any more than there's arguing with death. And soon, as I'm allowing my hair color to blend toward its natural state now, my patients will feel their way into our mutual aging a little bit differently when we face each other in the consulting room.

SPACIOUSNESS, STILLNESS, AND QUIET

A feeling of spaciousness is accompanying my aging. In my psychotherapy practice with patients, I notice that both the transference and the counter-transference have a little more room to breathe now that I'm older, and have been practicing for so long. I also sit with my patients with greater stillness now than I did years ago. And the stillness is *quieter* than before, enabling me to hear the patient's voice from this angle and that, its whispers, resonances, and melodies. When storms arise, I'm not washed away as I once was, though I can still get the breath knocked out of me. In the quiet, the patient's words can live their own life, with less interference from me now than before.

Over the years, psychotherapy and zazen have been my pathways into this spaciousness, stillness and quiet. Each discipline requires me to sit down and pay attention, and these seemingly simple practices create a powerful structure that contains and supports me. Each cuts down on extraneous distraction and stimulation, and each encourages the spirits of inquiry and love that are necessary in the face of difficulty. Each makes a space for the suffering that runs through this human life to express itself, in the midst of powerful personal and cultural denials of how difficult life is. These denials cannot be overcome by willpower, but only by paying attention, which, it turns out, can be thought of as a form of love.

Norman Fischer, Zen priest and poet, in his book *Taking Our Places*, makes these comments about the benefits of zazen, which I believe can be similarly said about psychotherapy: "Meditation practice is a powerful way of getting deeply in touch with your life at its most essential level . . . . Meditation practice makes it more possible for us to act out of our deepest, calmest, most accurate selves" (Fischer, 2003, pp. 108, 109).

Both psychotherapy and meditation practices support me in my effort to stay open, to remember how much I don't know. For example, I was sure I had a self. But sitting on my meditation cushion, I notice my tendency to gather up my experiences in a way that creates a *feeling* of a self. That self may seem to be located somewhere, but on looking closely I notice that that place is actually just a thought, or it's a place in my body where I hold my energy a certain way, or it's a collection of physical and energetic sensory experiences connected with the thoughts that are passing through what I think of as me. Experienced in this way, my self appears as an illusion in the larger field of consciousness. Over time, my concepts of "self" and "other" have become more complicated than they once were. The transformations we therapists witness in clinical life are their own teachings in emptiness and impermanence, in the illusory nature of the self, as they permit us to view the insubstantiality and changeability of the self despite our day-to-day feelings of continuity and identity.

When we become attuned to the subtlest aspects of our experience, and relax our grip on our ideas about things, we approach the transcendental. Over decades of practice I have noticed how intimately connected we are with our patients; at the deepest level there is no separation between life and life, heart and heart. Life moves through our clinical hours with its own truths, and our stories seem to speak for the generations who are making their appearances through our small selves. As I explore the nonlinear nature of time, it appears that we are healing, in our work, not only our own heart and the patient's heart today, but our past experiences and the hearts of our ancestors.

REFERENCES

Bromberg, D. (1998). *Standing in the spaces: Essays on clinical process, trauma and dissociation*. Hillsdale, NJ: The Analytic Press.

Ellman, J. (1996). Analyst and patient at midlife. *Psychoanalytic Quarterly, 65,* 353–371.

Fischer, N. (2003). *Taking our places*. New York, NY: HarperCollins.

Hanh, T. N. (2001). *Transformation at the base*. Berkeley, CA: Parallax Press.

Issacharoff, A. & Hunt, W. (1978). Beyond countertransference. *Contemporary Psychoanalysis, 14,* 241–310.

Stern, D. (2003). *Unformulated experience: From dissociation to imagination in psychoanalysis*. Hillsdale, NJ: The Analytic Press.

Unforeseen and Transformative: New Dimensions in the Third Quarter of My Life

AMITY PIERCE BUXTON

Founding Director of Straight Spouse Network, El Cerrito, California

Themes of the transformation marking the third quarter of my life were (a) an integration of non-Western philosophies and cultural traditions into my personal and professional perspective, (b) a deepening patience with the change process, (c) a recognition of the competing roles of personal accountability and context, (d) increasing internal energy and conceptualization power, and (e) realization of attitudinal shifts, physical and cognitive diminishment, altered coping styles, reordered priorities, and intimations of mortality that come with aging. My background is in teacher education for desegregating multiethnic schools. The changes I describe here were triggered by my husband's coming out as gay; my remarriage; my travels in Asia; explorations of science and metaphysics; founding the worldwide Straight Spouse Network to support, counsel, and educate straight spouses of gay, lesbian, bisexual, and transgender partners and their families; moving to a retirement community; and activism to achieve equality in society, especially within faith communities.

PRELUDE

I was already on the change track as the second half of my life began. I grew up on the East Coast, in a family who believed there was but one correct way to do or say anything, and with my own code that viewed compromise as a betrayal of integrity. At age 23 I found myself teaching at a unionized

Midwestern public high school. Two years later, I was teaching freshman English at a California state college to a class that included Korean War veterans and a language lab for prospective teachers who were immigrants or children of foreign-born parents. These experiences dealt a deathblow to any remaining notions of "only one way" and demolished the "safe" path of my childhood.

Changes continued as I earned an interdisciplinary PhD, married, and gave birth to a son in Paris and a daughter in San Francisco. At home, our children were being raised in a bilingual context: I conversed with them in French only, and my husband in English.

I continued teaching and coordinated curriculum for a university-based teacher education project. The project would help teachers desegregate elementary schools. Some of these schools were in a multiethnic urban district; others were in a suburban area where a Black-only district and a White-only district were going to merge. Next, I directed a center where teachers developed active learning materials and interdisciplinary units so that all children, irrespective of "differences," could learn and reach their full potential. Then, I became staff development coordinator for an urban multiethnic school district.

By the time I was 54, these experiences had made me keenly conscious of how individual and social changes take place. I observed the role that cultural context plays in how people live and think, the critical function of experience in one's learning, and the variations and untapped potential of humankind. Therefore, when my husband told me he was gay, after 25 years of marriage, I was stunned, yes, and also armed with skills needed to plunge into a more multileveled, complex world, where I would discover an even deeper core of commonalities alongside limitless differences and permeable boundaries, leading to where I am today at age 79.

UNFOLDING OF THE THIRD QUARTER

From age 54 to 79, a series of life and work experiences extended and deepened my strengths, knowledge, and awareness, through a cross-fertilization process.

Context, Complexity, Diversity

I tried to integrate the meaning of my gay husband's disclosure into my day-to-day life. I discovered and then devoured books, lectures, and workshops on metaphysical systems by which people in many cultures found meaning in life, from Native American to Sufi. I became ill with mononucleosis, the result of burning the candle at both ends as I tried to gain some sense of myself after my husband's unexpected revelation. During my recuperation, I read extensively, and among other books, I discovered *Siddhartha*,

Herman Hesse's (2000) account of the Buddha's life. Slowly, I began to discern the difference between "being" and "becoming" and recognized the kind of transformation that starts from within.

The nondualistic paradigms common to most of the non-Western, indigenous, or ancient cultures began to inform my daily life and later my counseling. My assumptions about gender and marriage were shattered. My moral compass and my belief system were in doubt as a result of my husband's turning out to be gay, turning out to not be a straight man. The binary view that categorizes events as true or false, good or evil, salvatory or damnable, could not explain why the person closest to me turned out to not be what he had presented to me as his identity and sexual orientation. What helped me understand the situation was the nondualism of Buddhism, Hinduism, Sufism, indigenous tribes, and medieval Christian and Jewish mysticism. Here were no answers, rather a new way to look at life's most profound questions. These teachings, embedded in their respective cultures, enabled me to form a wider view of the different ways people handle life's vicissitudes and forge belief systems.

Meanwhile, an organization of once-married gay fathers requested that I write a book about straight spouses so that they could better understand their straight wives. To gather information for the book, I interviewed straight wives and husbands, and also gay, lesbian, and bisexual individuals who were or had been in mixed-orientation marriages. The interviews, and the scant research literature available on the topic, revealed the painful struggles that precede a married gay person's disclosure, the interplay of the biological-chemical underpinnings, and environmental factors that form sexual orientations and the psychological, emotional, physical, and spiritual upheaval that a spouse's coming out causes for his or her straight spouse. Finding out the personal experience of these individual and relational crises extended my awareness of the layers of context and the complexity of factors involved in a married person's disclosure. The phenomenon of bisexuality itself opened my eyes further to the restrictiveness of a dualistic either/or way of viewing sexual orientation and the more productive potential of having a both/and perspective, the same nondichotomous perspective that my metaphysical exploration had fostered.

A second marriage to a journalist who shared my interest in nontraditional belief systems led to travel in Asia, Latin America, and the Middle East. There, I made direct contact with people living in cultures that I had never encountered in prior travels and learned about their daily and special ritual practices based on their diverse worldviews. These travels, and my reading in social science and philosophy, heightened my sense of the interconnectedness of people and of all aspects of the natural world.

In addition, living with a new husband gave me insight into the distinct dynamics in relationships and the unique ways in which different families interact. Each family has its own ethos and "rules" that members must navigate in order to feel that they belong. Within the ethos of their particular family, individuals work through their issues and become comfortable with their "truth." Now, with a stepfamily added to my family of two children and a former husband with whom I kept in close contact I learned a new pecking order, new relationship patterns, control centers, and new expectations for how one should act and interact.

Continuity and Change: Teaching and Learning

TEACHING AND COUNSELING

The publication of my book *The Other Side of the Closet: The Coming-Out Crisis for Straight Spouses* (Buxton, 1994) led me to found the Straight Spouse Network, an organization for providing peer support and research-based information to straight spouses and families. I continued in the role of teacher as I gave presentations on the impact on families of a spouse's coming out. I also found myself becoming a counselor as I talked and e-mailed with spouses through the network and facilitated a peer support group. As I counseled, all of the transforming experiences within my own life fed my work. I also kept adding to my technical knowledge of psychology, begun in undergraduate and graduate classes, through readings and workshops.

As I was asked to speak in more venues, I began to meet spouses of transgender mates and transgender men and women. The nonduality framework that I brought to these conversations and counseling experiences helped me to grasp the both/and nature of gender identity and expression that is inherent in transgenderism. This understanding deepened my grasp of distinctions between person and expression, between biological and assigned. I also came to understand more fully the need for congruence among the factors that comprise a person's self-concept or identity.

Continued research on and writing about straight spouses, mixed-orientation and trans/nontrans couples, and children in these families gradually shifted the focus of my social justice work. Once again, I was working as a change agent from within. However, this time my aim was to eliminate antigay and antitrans social and religious attitudes and to challenge societal expectations that heterosexual marriage is the sole acceptable form of marriage.

EMPATHY AND RELATIONSHIP

A surprising development enhanced both my personal life and professional practice. From listening to spouses' narratives and through the process of creating a new relationship with my second husband, I slowly increased my comprehension of the subtle factors at work in relationship-building.

I saw how these dynamics can shift the balance, either strengthening or weakening the relationship and the individuals therein; for example, codependence versus interdependence, or one-sided caregiving versus the mutual nurturance of each partner's autonomy.

Empathy was another area that grew stronger as I counseled spouses in mixed-orientation or trans/nontrans marriages. As a young woman, when I considered majoring in psychology I had feared I would be too sympathetic with clients and decided instead to become a teacher. I now discovered the practice of empathy as I helped spouses resolve their pressing needs and issues and reconfigure their lives. Gradually, I got beyond solely understanding their feelings and what they were thinking or feeling to what Paul Elken (2007) describes as compassionate empathy, where a person not only understands and senses the feelings of another but also "spontaneously moves to help them if needed."

Meanwhile, wisdom crept unannounced into my life through the very process of living more years. My passionate concern about people on the margins became tempered by a more informed understanding of the different contexts in which marginal groups live and the various ways individuals react to and cope with difficulties. Through my work, I became increasingly aware of the effects that ethnicity, sexual orientation, gender identity, and expression, age, location, socioeconomic class, belief system, educational level, occupation, and community of faith often have on an individual when making a life-changing decision. At the core of my continuing transformation lay a humbling realization of the "bottom line" nature of personal choice, the owning of one's problems and solutions, and greater patience with the slow process of change. Passionate activism was needed, yes, but also a deliberate plan of action based on comprehensive knowledge of the terrain.

Living With, and Learning From, Old People

Almost three years ago, another abrupt change in my personal life accelerated my awareness of the factors that underlie life's major decisions and actions. My husband has cerebellar ataxia and peripheral neuropathy, progressive neurological conditions. We realized we needed to move to a retirement community where medical assistance would be readily available. Living in community with women and men in their 80s, 90s, and 100s, many of whom had been highly productive in their fields as professors, scientists, clergy, and community leaders—and all but one older than I—has been enlightening and sobering.

Becoming part of the "community" has been a learning process. We live communally. Our late neighbor here introduced me to the communal concept the week we moved in. I've come to understand the communal concept as one in which the common good is the measure of what one does and doesn't do, and friendliness and service provide the fuel to keep the commonwealth alive and well. Not every resident accepts or understands the communal ethic. Thanks to my neighbor's mentoring, I have found the community concept to be a mellowing force, allowing me to focus my energy on clarifying what I need, value, and do as an individual and allowing me to contribute my talents to the commonwealth rather than seek power or fame within it.

Much more important than power or status has been the ready-made chance to learn from the more than one hundred people with whom I live and interact daily. Living within this ethnically diverse group continually illustrates the interplay between the universality of the physical and cognitive effects of aging and the diversity coping styles and attitudes. At dinner, we often eat with two history professors who supported the Free Speech student movement during the 1960s in Berkeley; now, without pomp or pride, they share their scholarly knowledge of previous presidents and compare them to what the United States government is doing now. Other times, we dine with another couple, a technology expert/community college professor and a seamstress, whose families separately escaped from Nazi Germany to South America, she to a life of poverty and no schooling from age 12 to her 20s when she came to San Francisco. They enthrall us with lively stories about Germany and Ecuador, debate current events with us, and make us laugh with their delicious sense of humor. The mellowing that comes with time and access to layers of memory is especially noticeable when talking with my Japanese-American friends who were in internment camps as children and yet seem to harbor no resentment.

Acceptance, and rising above immediate pain, is observable almost everywhere here. For example, I share reports and pictures of newly designed buildings from the *New York Times* with an architect; he in turn shares articles about Mormonism and the struggles of gay Mormons. Listening to his articulate words and watching his alert face, one would never know that he has had two shoulders replaced and a spinal surgery in the past three years. Then there is the former fireman, whose painful back causes him to walk with difficulty; still, he "works" the beverage table for events, smilingly serves the theme drink, whether it is champagne, hot buttered rum, or cider. Another, who has become totally deaf, is a woman who has developed areas of nonverbal creativity and community service. She creates three-dimensional "zipper paintings" (yes, entirely created out of discarded zippers) and also offers to hem residents' clothes. In exchange for these art pieces and useful services, she receives a few dollars that she donates to help fund resident programs, from music to filmed lectures from the Learning Company.

Relationship building surrounds me. Friendships are made between new arrivals and old-timers. Widows and widowers and the divorced find new companions, several since we have been here. Most connect unexpectedly. As one couple who married in their eighties, said, "No one was as surprised as we." Then there are the couples who have been married for over 50 years, clearly different from each other in temperament, the degree of physical impairment, and problem solving styles, but bonded by a shared history, mutual respect, and acceptance of the way things are, and, just as clearly, loving the person whose habits or foibles annoy them.

A shift of priorities comes with retirement and age. No longer in positions of prestige and power as leaders in their fields, my fellow residents use their talents to serve others in this community, with scarcely any reference to their former work as they caringly perform new tasks. If asked, they will recount their stories, not to boast but just to contribute to the conversation. For example, the former physicist who worked at Los Alamos brushes aside any reference to that period of his life as he runs the Make and Mend shop where he fixes household items that break or break down, from lamps to jewelry cabinets, or makes stands or bins to order. He and his crew, too, give the dollar paid for their services to fund the resident programs.

At the same time, there are many in their 80s and early 90s who continue their outside work. One woman volunteers weekly at a hospital; the former fund-raiser who lived in Brazil now tutors Brazilian students attending the University of California; the doctor mentors medical students; and the former telephone worker reads weekly with immigrant children at an elementary school in the nearby town where she used to live.

Observing human nature mellowing with age provides me with models of acceptance marked with a curious kind of joy. I especially resonated with a woman, now dead, who had three husbands and, confined to a wheel chair, emanated a joyous sprit each time she spoke, whether about daily events, her family, or her past experiences as a singer.

As I marvel and enjoy these new friends, it is sobering to watch them and others become more frail with each passing week. It is unsettling to watch my husband's increasing loss of balance and difficulty in reading and remembering, while I am totally blown away by how he accepts these losses with equanimity and humor. I gasp each time I see yet another In Memoriam sign by the elevator. Today it was the former Foreign Service officer who had lived in China and Brazil for many years. After the shock, I reminded myself how fortunate I was to know him. With each death, however, I am more and more conscious of the reality of the imminent, though unknown, time that my own capacity to produce or to fulfill my constantly multiplying goals will end, and, of course, that my life itself will end.

On a practical level, this awareness of the effects of aging has prompted me to take better care of myself physically. I pay attention to how I walk so I don't fall (I have fallen twice with serious effects), do strength exercises regularly, and set priorities of what I do, say, write, and plan, so that I can live long enough to fulfill all that needs to be done.

Life and Work at 79

At age 79, I have no intention of stopping work for some time. Assessing what I bring to my work and life, I find that most of my old habits of perception and behavior are still central, while some have been reinforced or expanded. In addition, several new practices have replaced those that were ill-suited in certain circumstances or ineffective anywhere. These continuities and changes (plus changes that will be made to fit new circumstances and understandings) will enable me to meet my hopes for the last quarter of my life.

Personal Strengths, Priorities, Perspectives, and Practices

My spiritual and metaphysical explorations strengthened several of my natural inclinations. These strengths include sensitivity to others' needs, craving for balance while in the grips of intense feeling, creativity, reflection and introspection, and flexibility. Each of these elements has become stronger in my life and work. All of them enabled me to survive and grow as a person after my husband came out.

Simultaneously, my experience and observation of individual and social change caused a shift in my priorities, in both my life and my work. Building bridges of understanding between people has now become as important to me as helping people individually. Collaboration, which I learned long ago on my high school sports teams, brings about more effective outcomes than individualism. The seeds of this recognition were planted during my involvement as an ally with the civil rights and gay movements, working collaboratively to desegregate schools and curriculum. My recognition is validated as I observe how peer support and help enables spouses to resolve a disparate array of issues.

A related and completely new development is my patient trust in the healing, regenerative, and reconfiguration potential of human beings. I am more aware that, for this potential to become actual, people must be given support, reality-based information, and tools, and be encouraged to take individual responsibility.

SPIRITUAL PRACTICES: CONNECTION, THE PRESENT CHANGE, AND TRANSCENDENCE

This perspective, which has transformed the core of my life and my counseling work, has been forged primarily from the non-Western philosophies and mystical religions. I continue to stay in touch with them through readings and workshops. Through these teachings, I recognize the interconnectedness of all elements in life and the world—the Taoists concept of yin and yang that need to be balanced; the oneness principle in Hinduism, that each of us is an individual drop of water that comprises one ocean; the Native American concept of the circle of life, at one with the earth and Great Spirit. My appreciation and resonance with these complementary concepts from different cultures is accompanied by my growing interest in and awareness of the nonphysical, unseen yet felt "energies" that permeate my experience.

The Eastern practice of focusing on the present is also important to me. Discerning and handling what is happening now—my husband's illness, straight spouses' needs, developing community in my new home, and my spiritual growth—form my main task and color my guidance of the spouses I counsel. While I continue to take a long-range view of life and work, through reflection, I know that it is not helpful to focus on the past or future, neither of which one can control.

The Buddhist and Hindu recognition of the constancy of change—"this too will pass," the good as well as the bad—has helped me get through painful times (whether I was in a semicoma in India or dealing with a relative's alcoholism). Now, it helps me deal with daily challenges of living in an institutional setting and assists me in calming the urgency that many spouses feel when they are mired in pain and grief. "Slowly, slowly" is a mantra I share with many of them, whether by e-mail or in person. I am learning to view their suffering, and my own, as part of the ongoing nature of life rather than a measure of whether we are good or bad. This helps me, and them, see that how one deals with the pain and grief is what matters most.

From Sufism and mysticism, the notion of transcendence—the intimation that true reality lies behind appearances—helps me and, in turn, through my sharing, helps many straight spouses begin to trust our inner truth. The loss of trust in one's inner truth is part of the trauma that straight spouses suffer after their partners come out. That trust must be recovered in order to take the leap of faith needed to step forward. Akin to this is the Toltec idea that we each have our own "dream" picture of the world in our heads and we are the only ones who know what it is. Based on this inner information, to which only each individual has access, the Toltec wisdom names four principles for honoring and capitalizing on that knowledge: do not make assumptions, do not take things personally, be impeccable with your word, and do your best. Implementing this wisdom has enabled me to weather turmoil in my personal and professional life. Affirmed by my personal experience, these four principles have also helped the people who I counsel restore confidence and trust, even while they feel hurt, their assumptions are shattered, their trust has been broken, and they feel like failures.

PRACTICES FOR PERSONAL AND PROFESSIONAL HEALING

The Hindu dictum to act in a way that is right, rather than for reward or honor, has made me impervious to criticism within my marriage or family, in my new community, and in the Straight Spouse Network organization. In turn, this message informs what I say to straight spouses and seems to help them reconfigure their own moral code and integrity. Forgiving my gay husband was done not as act of judging, or assuming authority for his absolution, or as a way to gain approval for doing the right thing. Rather, it was done from the belief that forgiveness is a powerful way to release one's own pain or anger through loving compassion for oneself and the other person.

Practices based on my experience help spouses do their own healing work. One of the most powerful is a ritual that I still do from time to time. In this healing ceremony, I burn something that symbolizes a part of my past as a way to let go of it or to cleanse myself of regrets. Some people I counsel resonate with this practice, finding that it helps them let go and look forward. Another rite is a "hoping ceremony" in which I write a hope or future vision on a piece of paper, burn it, and watch the smoke rise into the sky. A third rite celebrates the good in what needs to be left behind, an act that both honors and releases with acceptance. The last day that I spent moving our things from our former house to the retirement community I built a fire in our fireplace and gave a toast with a glass of red wine, to the happy time my husband and I spent there. And then I watched the flames finally go out, before I said the final "good-bye."

Heightened Sense of History

In addition to non-Western philosophies, a heightening of a sense of history affects me as I approach 80. This sense of history came vividly into the present as I sifted through my personal and professional belongings in order to decide which to take to the retirement community and which to give away. (I'm still making those decisions about piles of packed boxes.)

The sense of history became vivid in 2007 when I decided to turn the leadership of Straight Spouse Network over to a younger generation. Even now, watching President Obama's election ceremonies, I am keenly conscious of the ongoingness of the social movements of which I was and am still a part. With fewer years ahead of me to be part of these movements, I am concerned about what will happen next, particularly to support and inspire people in marginal groups who have not yet profited from the social changes: the poor, the immigrants, the imprisoned, and the ill. Will I live to see the changes?

Faith-Based Activism

My own crisis of faith as a Catholic following my first husband's disclosure is mirrored in the stories of many spouses whose faith-based beliefs were shaken by our gay, lesbian, bisexual, or transgender partner's disclosure. The more conservative the faith community, the more of a challenge because of the guilt and fear of damnation of the gay, lesbian, bisexual, or transgender partner and the stigma often transferred to the straight spouse and children. Both spouses struggle to integrate personal experience and religious doctrine. Some leave their church or temple and find a more welcoming congregation, while many others cut off any religious connection except their personal faith, and some lose that too.

My own faith crisis was resolved through readings, prayer, workshops, experience of the non-Western belief systems, and through my new husband's interest in spirituality and membership in the Unitarian Universalist church, which I joined and attended, while still going to mass each week. I came to recognize that love and truth were the core principles for leading my life and for dealing with restrictive antigay religious doctrines. Focusing on love and truth as bottom line principles, in turn, enabled me to help some spouses leaven their faith-based views about gay, lesbian, bisexual, and transgender persons. As I gradually found myself assuming a pastoral role with spouses coping with the faith. I smiled, recalling that after my husband came out, I had temporarily thought of becoming a Lutheran so that I could be an ordained priest and thereby be able to minister.

Now I am becoming more of a religious activist. I am writing, meeting, and joining leadership groups working in their communities of faith to achieve acceptance of gay, lesbian, bisexual, and transgender persons, the legality of same-sex marital unions, and the practice of truth and love, which I believe lie at the heart of all religions. I have just accepted a board position for the Catholic Association for Lesbian and Gay Ministries.

SENSITIVITY TO CONTEXT

As I counsel people of different ethnicities, echoes come from my work in education during the 1960s and 1970s. Like the public school community people with whom I worked, each ethnic and racial group of spouses has its own set of concerns based on culture of origin. Concerns often stem from concepts of family, sexuality, and marriage and ideas about gay, lesbian, bisexual, or transgender people held by their particular racial or ethnic group. Many African Americans are closely involved in family-oriented church communities where homosexuality is viewed as an "abomination," causing many black gay and bisexual men to stay closeted, often engaging in same-sex behavior "on the down low," while the congregants deny their being gay or pray for their conversion. In Asian cultures, too, denial and hiding are common, and spouses choose to rely on their own resources to deal with their partner's disclosure rather than reveal their situation to professionals. Hispanics tend to have strong family ties also, making it difficult for gay spouses to admit their orientation and for straight spouses to tell anyone about the disclosure. Out of concern that the Straight Spouse Network was not addressing issues confronting spouses in these marginal groups, I initiated an outreach project for underserved spouses a year ago.

Counseling: An Amalgam

As a result of these changes in my life and the way I coped with them, my counseling work now is an amalgam of the philosophical, psychological, and cultural concepts that were slowly integrated into my practice. Simultaneously, the experience of counseling spouses for the past 20 years has given me a wealth of concrete examples and has given me time to hone techniques that validate the strengths and potential of counselees so that they can discover they are able to heal and transform themselves and their lives. This practice of confirming their capabilities, and illustrating with specific examples, has proved to be more empowering for my counselees than unspecified praise or general suggestions (which characterized my approach in my years of teaching).

My eyes are constantly on the lookout for clues to the contexts in which a spouse is embedded. At the ready are knowledge and concepts that might help a particular spouse resolve concerns, manage emotions, and reformulate a personal philosophy so that they can reconfigure their lives as I did mine, not taking the same path as I took but honoring the same process. In one way, my approach has become more like that of a doctor diagnosing the common issues: which is most troublesome to a particular spouse? Which is the spouse's overriding emotion? What is her or his greatest source of strength?

Empowerment

The goal of empowering spouses drives my work, while I remain conscious of the time needed for them to reach the last stage of transformation. I need to keep reminding them how long it takes to heal; cope; clarify wants, needs, and values; and resolve their concerns while readjusting their moral compass and formulating a realistic belief system. Healing can start only after they face, acknowledge, and accept the new reality. Also, I clarify, they cannot "rebuild" their lives. Rather, they need to reconfigure their belief system based on the new reality. Then they can start afresh.

Facing a spouse counselee is daunting. Rather than the expert-learner interaction of the teaching I used to do, counseling is now a shared experience. I bring knowledge and wisdom gained from experience and study, and the spouse brings his or her sense of personal capabilities and experience and gradually takes responsibility for choosing action to meet his or her goals. The process is similar to teaching in that it is up to the learner whether or not to learn. However, as a wise man I dated in the postdisclosure period told me, "We find our own teachers."

Few strategies in my work remain intact from my teaching years. Most have been expanded to include more directive guidance and more information to enable and empower spouses to implement their decisions. Rather than the cheerleading approach that I used to take, I now offer specific illustrations of the effective things they have done and why they are effective and whatever information they need to take further steps. Still other strategies are freshly designed.

The most essential tool in my practice is two-way communication, including asking questions, validating, educating, and listening, all four intertwined. Listening is the practice that I have expanded most. Two-way communication involves enabling the counselee to talk while I listen, and my questioning or probing while they listen. I am less likely now to focus on the spouse's presenting problem, form an interpretation, impose my sense of what the issue is, and/or to suggest a resolution based on my and other spouses' reported experience. Rather, I find myself waiting for or asking for a spouse's own interpretation or resolution, knowing that it is probably more accurate than mine.

I strengthened several strategies by adding key elements that helped me after my first husband came out. During my own therapy, in several times of crisis or crossroads, the therapist mirrored or validated my feelings, attitudes, and capabilities and took a questioning approach that caused me to identify my own issues, needs, wants, and values. Using this model, I validate spouses' worth and strength and also point out alternative possibilities, based on glimpses I catch of their special qualities while listening to them. Identifying counselees' sources of strength or underlying concerns has more motivating power when I explain why that virtue or concern is important or what relevance it has to their situation.

Somewhat similar, my questioning put the onus on the spouses to put into words realizations about themselves that they never knew they had. Querying them about various aspects of a situation and then guiding them to ask questions of themselves often elicits one or more self- discoveries and usually leads to their making plans of action to resolve issues and move forward.

The Value of Time

Underlying all of the strategies, giving spouses the gift of time is what I have learned to value most highly—time to figure out what their issues really are. I make explicit that time is itself a process that cannot be hurried or short-circuited and explain that letting time move at its natural pace allows for trial-and-error testing of alternatives, self-examination, discovering new insights, eliminating unproductive habits, and absorbing new experiences. All of these activities, I explain, are the ingredients needed to make the examined, integrated, and constructive life decisions that will enable them to reconfigure their lives in a positive direction. "Slowly, slowly" is a mantra I often use.

Multiple outcomes are possible for these spouses, and their issues take much longer to resolve than any of them expects or wants. A spouse's reconfiguration of his or her self-concept, moral compass, trust, sense of self worth, integrity and belief system cannot be hurried, and the results cannot be predicted.

Just as I slowed down in my own life to keep pace with the process of change, so I have slowed down how I work with spouses. Now, I no longer quickly figure out what a spouse needs, but rather guide him or her over a number of months to move in a forward direction while I maintain a positive tone, contribute constructive information, and communicate compassionate, action-related empathy, all the time reminding them to take their time. Reminding them of the slowness of this process is critical, since most partners or families keep saying, "Get on with it. It's time to move on!"

AT THE THRESHOLD OF THE UNKNOWN FUTURE

Where I Live Informs My Work

My valuing of time, and the importance of taking one's time when faced with life's challenges, developed through tracking straight spouses' transformative work, through my research on strategies for staying married after a spouse came out (the most frequently mentioned was "taking our time"), and, most recently, through observing how older persons in this residential community conduct the last years of their lives.

Just as I experienced a slight but profound shift in my perception of how best to live when I was in India, so there has been another small but profound shift in my outlook in the three years I have been in this retirement community. Rather than striving for achievement, I find myself preoccupied with understanding the nature of people and of consciousness, and with communicating whatever wisdom I gain, through my work.

This deep change took place unnoticed as I listened to the life stories of my fellow residents, observed their patient acceptance of the personal consequences of life's passage as their bodies become more fragile and their memories less clear. I am constantly struck by the way their inner core sparkles, in the eyes or the smiles of those who care for one another, or when they articulate their opinions on a current affairs issue such as the environmental crisis or change in president.

Even so, having to deal with deaths of people, some new friends, whose long experience I value and whose wisdom feeds my energies, has battered my sense of invincibility and my "all will be well" outlook. I shudder, cringe when fellow residents jokingly refer to where we live as "a holding place." Seeing the reality of death, however, makes me crave even more strongly for as much time as can be given me and the ability to use it wisely and efficiently.

Placing Myself in the Generations

The difference between the kind of counseling I do now and the more teacherly and nondirective counseling of 25 years ago becomes clearer daily as I work with a younger generation of peer counselors in the Straight Spouse Network. Many (though not all) are quick to judge or advise, not allowing time for a spouse to sort out issues and resolve problems. They tend to seek results sooner rather than later. In some cases, they give so much of themselves that they lose sight of their objective, which is helping spouses help themselves heal and grow in understanding.

Of course, the younger volunteer peer counselors have other responsibilities in their lives that I no longer share. Most have paid jobs, do the constant work of parenting, and many are trying to make ends meet as single parents. In contrast, I have time to watch counselees progress patiently. Yes, I am a caregiver to my husband, yet I have no other responsibilities for parenting, home repairs, or earning a salary.

In addition, I bring to my practice a quarter of a century of dealing with personal crises, transforming my life, traveling, reading, studying, researching, writing, and doing groundbreaking professional work, and I have amassed a wealth of wisdom gained from interaction with diverse cultures and colleagues. I also bring a lifelong habit of reflective introspection, which grew stronger through my personal journey after my first husband's disclosure. If I were a Hindi male at this point in my life cycle, I would leave my family to live as a wandering, ascetic teacher. As an American female, I can live with my husband, my adult children nearby, and counsel a largely ignored group of people with profound needs.

Finally, the spiritual and experiential developments that made me who I am and what I do today are now fueled by an ever-growing awareness of the potency of forgiveness, gratitude, and love—perhaps the most precious gifts of an older age.

As for Me and My Journey

As I continue in the last third of my life, living and working both enrich me. Compared to 25 years ago, I see my own needs and those of individual spouses and couples as more complex (because I know more) and, at the same time, more simple to resolve (because I am wiser). For both insights, I am grateful.

As for me and my journey, I now have more humility, peace, hope, and faith in the process of simply living. Yet challenges and questions abound. Being in a retirement community where I will "live the rest of my life" is a daunting concept to internalize. It means that the frontiers for my writing and social justice projects are no longer limitless. Every moment must count; none can be wasted. I clearly have to set priorities and accept the fact that the piles of sewing and ironing and artwork around the apartment may never get done.

Strangely, or perhaps not so strangely, as my body now looks more and more old and wrinkled—everywhere!—my physical energy has not decreased and my mental energy has increased. Whether dancing on a Florida beach at a drumming circle or exploring the kinds of energies that Carlos Castaneda writes about, or writing my own articles, poems, or responses to spouses, my energy seems boundless. My interest in metaphysics and in learning about and practicing non-Western philosophies has grown exponentially. All of these interests have been nourished by interaction with several spouses with similar proclivities and through serendipitous readings. These resources affirm that the world is full of opportunities to further my personal work. Right now, ongoing counseling and writing give me tremendous satisfaction. For continuing to be capable—able to live, act, think, and express myself fully in these ways, whether in words or dance or art or music or dreams—I thank God daily.

Since I am an only child and neither of my adult children has children, it could be that my dying will end the family line started by the ancestor who came to America on the second sailing of the Mayflower. Questions abound from this thought: Does this mean it's the end of our family? The Chinese say that a person keeps living as long as some survivor remembers that person. How might my memory of family history be preserved, once my children die? Whom would it help anyway? Who would be interested? What archives can I leave regarding my work, and who would put it to use?

Whatever the answers ultimately are, I feel a strong compulsion to write all I can about my life, for my children and for the professional community, about all of the social religious, political, economic, psychological, and cultural factors that impact families when a spouse comes out. Someone will surely want to read that.

The core questions for me at this juncture of my life are: Of what value is wisdom that comes with age? To whom is it of value—only the person who has become wise? If the wisdom of age is of value to others, how can one impart it so that it can help those who survive us to create more enriched lives for themselves and help our professional successors to generate more effective counseling practices? I pray that the answers will come and my energies last long enough to create such a legacy.

REFERENCES

Buxton, A. (1994). *The other side of the closet: The coming-out crisis for straight spouses and families*. New York: John Wiley & Sons.
Elken, P. (2007). Conversation with Paul Elken. Retrieved June 12, 2007, from www.DanielColeman.com.
Hesse, H. (2000). *Siddhartha*. Boston, MA: Shambhala Books.

The Therapist's Illness As an Opportunity in the Clinical Hour

SANDRAH HENRY

The Laure Center, San Francisco, California

Our subjective experience of aging will have an impact on the cocreation of the therapeutic relationship. As therapists enter the last third of life, they need to anticipate possible disruptions to their practice due to increased physical vulnerability, and they need to plan for these disruptions. This may require confronting narcissistic defenses and denial. Professional resources are available to assist with the pragmatic steps needed for continuity of patient care. Viewing her clinical work through the lens of intersubjective theory, the author shares her own experience with a life-threatening illness. She describes the impact it had on her relationship with one patient and how it was possible for the patient to find considerable therapeutic value in her response to the therapist's illness. The therapist's clinical decision to self-disclose information about her diagnosis is considered from an intersubjective perspective.

One of the major side effects of aging is increased physical vulnerability and an amplified sense of the nearness of death. Some of us are fortunate to maintain excellent health well into old age, but some degree of physical and cognitive change is to be expected. From an intersubjective perspective, we know that everything we experience—and our feelings and attitude about what we experience—impacts the ever-changing relational field between the therapist and the patient. This is true, whether our patients are consciously aware of the changes we are experiencing or not and regardless of how we as therapists are dealing with these changes.

We are all vulnerable to illness and disability throughout our lives, but the longer we are alive, the more our vulnerability increases. I have spoken with many therapists regarding their feelings about their own aging process, their physical and cognitive vulnerabilities, and their thoughts about how these impact their work. I've also asked them about what provisions they have made for their practices in the event of sudden death or serious illness. For the most part, the therapists I spoke with seemed unaware of these concerns, or perhaps were even in denial about them.

Given that everything in the intersubjective dyad—spoken and unspoken, conscious and unconscious—is brought into the room and shapes and guides the therapeutic process, I believe that it is imperative for us, as therapists, to confront our most deeply held fears, so we are prepared to guide our patients wherever they need to go. We are able to take our patients only as deeply as we have ventured into our own psyche. It is important that we break our denial regarding our vulnerabilities.

For those of us in private practice, a common belief seems to be that we will continue to work into old age. We may see this as an advantage for our profession because we bring years of experience and an advantage to ourselves because we have a venue in which to remain vital and generative. On the other hand, sometimes the decision to remain in practice is predicated on a financial vulnerability that private practice clinicians face. Being self-employed, we have had to plan for our own retirement or possible disability without any assistance from an employer. We may not be as prepared financially as someone who has spent her career in an agency or corporation. The anxiety about this financial vulnerability may very well be split off, or left unacknowledged, yet this concern will enter into the cocreated intersubjective field.

THE AGING THERAPIST IN THE INTERSUBJECTIVE FIELD

Working within a relational psychology model, we are called on to acknowledge and consider the impact of our aging on the therapeutic dyad. From this theoretical perspective, all healing occurs in relationship. This model holds that, once the therapist and client come together, the notion of objective reality becomes obsolete. The only reality that exists is that which is a result of the interplay between both individuals' subjective experience. The work of therapy takes place in this interplay and in the examination of it. Through this process, patients become aware of their unconscious framework and the limitations that they place on their relationships and connections with others. The process allows the patient to bring these principles into consciousness, thus expanding and broadening their perceptions of themselves and the world around them.

From this perspective, it is a given that the patient is impacted by her reaction to the therapist's changing body and health. Likewise, we are impacted by our patients' health and aging process. With all the myths and stereotypes associated with aging one can imagine what thoughts and feelings exist in the intersubjective field if the therapist encounters health problems that result in physical changes, decreased energy or vitality, and/or mobility impairment.

In addition, as one ages, it is inevitable that death comes into the consulting room. How often does this become part of the dialogue between patient and therapist? As we get older, the universal theme of loss is always close at hand. We need to be able to speak about the unspeakable.

Planning

Therapists are accustomed to working with their patients through the vicissitudes of life (albeit with varying degrees of skill). At the same time, therapists are often not accustomed to dealing with events in their own lives that take them, emotionally and sometimes physically, away from their clients. An illness always changes one's perspective on oneself and on one's life, and this change in perspective takes place for both the one diagnosed and for those close to her. Illness strips away defenses and privacy. It is hard to hide one's physical illnesses or limitations from patients.

I have been deeply affected by Ann Steiner's work, which deals with the therapist's physical vulnerabilities, physical illness, and end of life issues. She has created a "living will" and plans for one's practice in the event of sudden death, terminal illness, or extended absence due to a personal emergency. She shares her own story, in which she had to take over her father's long-term psychotherapy practice when he was diagnosed with a terminal illness. That experience prompted her to develop a step-by-step model for therapists to create their own emergency response system and "private practice will," complete with sample letters, answering machine messages, and forms. She urges people to come together as teams rather than create their emergency response system on their own because it can be emotionally overwhelming for therapists to confront these issues. Steiner has written a letter to her clients that will be sent out in the event of her sudden death or unforeseen absence. She has designated transition therapists who are colleagues, but not close friends to be available to help the patients through the period of death and eventually on to referral to new therapists. She has written a message she wants to have on her answering machine in the event of her sudden death. Steiner's publication *The Therapist's Professional Will: A Complete Guide*, an enhanced compact disc, can be ordered through her Web site: www.drsteiner.net.

An Example of Profound Vulnerability in the Therapy

All of this came to life for me when I experienced a major disruption in my practice as a result of an illness. This illness caused me to be away from my practice for a month, without prior notice to my clients.

I had never really considered the possibility that I would have a life-threatening illness. I held the irrational belief that, since I had already dealt with a serious chronic illness earlier in my life and was currently in remission, this made me immune to any other serious disease. In addition to my "immunity," I had no family history of breast cancer, I was physically active, and ate mostly an organic vegetarian diet. I had regular mammograms and did monthly self-examinations. My partner found the lump seven months after a regularly scheduled mammogram. I had actually felt something a few months before and "forgot" to have it checked out because it wasn't very noticeable. When I first saw my surgeon, she thought that it was probably a cyst, because it didn't feel hard like most breast tumors. It turned out to be stage three cancer with lymph node involvement.

With cancer diagnoses, everything happens so fast. It was a whirlwind from discovery to treatment. I wasn't used to the urgency and the need to put myself first. I had to drop everything, including my work. I found that I wanted to isolate myself from everyone except my family and my very close friends. I did not want to talk to my patients or deal with their anxiety. During the two weeks from discovery to full diagnosis, I worried about how everyone would be affected if my disease had progressed to a stage where death was imminent. I felt overwhelmed. I did not have a "will" or crisis team set up to deal with this crisis. I didn't even have an updated will for myself. I had been thinking about drafting a will for myself and my practice for a long time, I just never got around to doing it. This meant that I needed to contact my patients myself, and deal with their responses, at a time when I could barely deal with my own. I had to make decisions about what I would tell them. I felt an added heaviness, knowing that I was abandoning my patients with no plan for them in my absence and not certain when I would feel well enough to return to work. I had to develop a plan and talk to colleagues about my patients, when I didn't want to have to take care of anyone. Needless to say, it was more than I could really handle.

I was fortunate to be able to be able to work, off and on, throughout my cancer treatment. People would tell me I was "heroic" for working, but it was a necessity for me. I had great health insurance through my job, but it was only a part-time job, and I depended on my private practice income in order to meet my expenses. In addition, I didn't feel right about abandoning my patients. I was torn, wished that I felt more able to choose freely whether to continue working and felt envious of people I met who were able to take a leave from their jobs in order to go through the treatment from start to finish. There were times that I could not work, due to nausea or fatigue. Other times, working provided a relief from focusing on myself.

What I did not anticipate was the profound opportunity that my newly experienced vulnerability provided in my relationships with my patients. One of my patients, Sue, was actively suicidal at the time of my diagnosis. I was diagnosed on November 2, and she had a tentative suicide date planned for late November, after her 45th birthday. I had seen Sue for many years. She is a survivor of profound childhood abuse. She is also bipolar, with treatment-resistant depression despite a complicated medication regimen. Her life has become more and more difficult over the years. When I first began working with her, she was a legal secretary in one of the most prestigious law firms in the country. She was finishing her bachelor's degree while working full time. She maintained a relationship with her parents, despite their continued emotional abuse. Sue had made a serious suicide gesture only weeks after first seeing me, when her partner broke off the relationship, right after her therapist of three years had gone on an unexpected leave of absence and referred her to me. The abandonment was too much for her. She made the suicide gesture, and we agreed that she needed to be hospitalized.

Now I am going to jump forward eleven years in our relationship. Sue is now on Social Security Disability, has cut off contact with her parents, is about to turn 45, and has a suicide contract with herself that if she doesn't get some relief from her almost-constant depression, she won't live another year. I am very worried. I am using every possible thing I can think of to discourage the plan. I am consulting everyone I know about my concerns, my clinical work, and my countertransference.

Abandonment, as I said, is her major issue. When she was about five years old, and rocking in the back seat of the car (which she did to soothe herself), her parents pulled the car over and put her out, telling her that they were going to leave her there because she was driving them crazy with her rocking. They actually drove off and left her, although they eventually came back. There was always the threat that they were going to give her to an orphanage if she talked back or was bad "one more time." This was the tenor of her childhood.

Now I am sick and feeling like I can't handle the stress of containing her depression. I can't keep her afloat when I feel like I'm drowning. Yet I feel I can't abandon her while she is barely holding onto herself. I decide to meet with her and tell her about my diagnosis. She is shocked and devastated by my news. She struggles with an ultimate fear of abandonment: death. What if I am to die and leave her? I worry that she might decide that she should go ahead and commit suicide because I might die soon anyway.

Instead, she begins to focus on my needs. She wants to know what I feel. I decide to tell her I'm scared, but that I'm trying to take things a day at a time. I tell her that I am using the same strategies to reduce my anxiety that she and I have worked on for years. I tell her that I will see her as often as possible over the months of my treatment but that I might have to cancel at the last minute, as I won't be able to predict how I will be feeling during chemo and radiation. Sue decides to go to a support group for family and friends of people with cancer. She tells me that she really wants to do something to help me, and I respond that what would help me the most would be if she would give up her suicide plan and in fact give up suicide as an escape altogether. She tells me that she wants to do that, for me and for her. She says that she can't think about ending her life when I am fighting so hard to keep my own.

Over the next six months of our work together, Sue began to make real changes in her life. She began implementing action that she had been unwilling to do prior to my diagnosis. She was utilizing techniques and strategies to confront her anxiety head on. She began to explore the spiritual side of herself by building an altar for me in her home. She lit candles every day and began to pray, even though she had an aversion to prayer and referred to herself as a "recovering Catholic." She began reading books on mindfulness meditation that I had suggested to her in the past. She made great movement.

My suffering allowed her to turn her attention outward. She had someone she could actively care for. By helping herself, she felt that she was helping me, that I wouldn't worry about her, and therefore my stress would be reduced. I was surprised at both her agency and her ability to draw on the work that we had done over the years, to help me in crisis. She brought me things that she thought I might like to eat, when nothing tasted good. She gave me a healing candle and socks to keep my feet warm in the hospital. She sent me funny cards and loaned me comedies from her video collection, a collection that I had encouraged her to build for herself over the years to help with her depression. She wanted to be important in my recovery and used my illness as a metaphor for finding meaning in her own life. My vulnerability ignited a spark in her that she didn't even know that she had. Her love for me inspired her to find meaning in her life, even if it wasn't what she wanted her life to be. Her shame decreased dramatically.

As I've said, I was fortunate to be able to work, off and on, through my illness. If I had been forced to abruptly end my practice or had chosen not to work at all during my illness the scenario would have played out quite differently. She would have felt shut out and deeply hurt if I had chosen to withhold my diagnosis from her. I feel that it would have been such an empathic breach that it might have been impossible to repair.

THE WORK

The power of the intersubjective field, when the therapist can fearlessly confront her own denial about mortality, physical vulnerability, and aging, is clearly displayed in this case. Our own process of aging and facing death deeply enhances the client's work. Bringing existential issues directly into the therapy deepens the therapeutic exchange and allows the therapist and patient to sit together in the knowledge that there will be inevitable losses. It encourages to us to keep our hearts open and be willing to face whatever is to come. This paradox leads to an appreciation for each other and can lead us to pay attention to our need to live in the present.

I am the kind of therapist who believes that the authentic use of self is one of the most important aspects of the therapeutic process. I am not advocating that we begin talking to clients about our anticipated illnesses or death secondary to aging. I am advocating that we talk to ourselves and our colleagues about them so that we can deal with clients more effectively, if and when the need arises. I also think that dealing more directly with ourselves and in our therapeutic communities will open us up to the shared experiences that life brings to every one of us.

Who Am I Now? Using Life Span Theories in Psychotherapy in Late Adulthood

VALORY MITCHELL

California School of Professional Psychology at Alliant University, San Francisco, California

Although academic and clinical psychology do not often embrace, lifespan developmental constructs and theories can enrich the process of psychotherapy. Particularly in the last third of life, when social institutions and societal expectations provide less guidance and constraint, access to understandings about the lifespan may be especially useful. A life structure model of 20-year eras and periods of stability and evaluation/transformation can bring structure when life appears amorphous. Recognition of the ways that people of different ages experience time, and lifetime, can increase empathy and promote client's understanding of their own changes. Three dimensions of development—the ethic of care, the acquisition of integrity, and the building of an individuated and mature ego—can bring increased depth, vitality, fullness, and enjoyment to the last third of life. Therapists' ability to detect and articulate their client's developmental needs and process can enhance the work and further client's growth.

About half a lifetime ago, I was a graduate student, working on a longitudinal study of the lives of 140 women. At that time (1978), psychology had seemed to suddenly discover adult development; new theories emerged, and studies were funded.

I found the idea of lifespan development fascinating. It was as though all of us were, without our knowing it, being carried along on the current of a river—the river of life. We had all been born, we would all die, and in between the river flowed. Not that every journey is the same; each is unique. But the further we get from the particulars of a life, the deeper we look below the surface of the water, the more we can recognize patterns and forces at work.

Parts of the river have maps, and a language, to describe them. As therapists, we know the power of language, of the ability to name and to witness. There is a magic in being able to name the changing flows and currents, the shallows and deeps that one is likely to encounter as the river moves along. And there is even more magic in seeing it as a whole, the entire span of the life span, in its completeness—and in its ultimate mystery.

I have spent my professional life as both a psychotherapist and an academic, and I am painfully aware of the lack of contact and communication between these two arms of psychology. This is sad, because when arms work together in an embrace, something wonderful can happen. Over 30 years later I am still fascinated by conceptions of lifespan development and I have found that some lifespan developmental ideas can enrich the experience of therapy, and this is especially so in the largely uncharted territory of the last third of life.

I will describe a few of these ideas—the importance of the regularly changing life structure, life as time, and three major psychological developments that give meaning and shape to the last third of life: the ethic of care, integrity, and the mature ego. I will offer some examples from my clinical work to illustrate how these ideas come to life in therapy.

THE STRUCTURE OF THE LIFE COURSE

In early life (at least in the industrialized countries), we live within a set of culturally legitimated, closely age-graded structures. We go through each grade at school, and then (often, though not always) to college as our transition into the adult world. Once beyond the institution of school, we may drift or experiment a bit during our 20s, but most of us will have charted our course and made commitments, usually to relationships/family and to work, by our early thirties. These commitments have been called "social clock projects" (Helson, Mitchell, & Moane, 1984) because, in every society, these projects are socially valued, and because we have an inner "clock" to tell us whether we have begun them "too early," "late," or "on time" according to the norms of our culture, class, and moment in history. For most of us, our early and middle adult years are largely shaped by our involvement in these projects, to which we devote most of our time, energy, and concern.

As we approach late adulthood, however, we begin to look on our projects from a different perspective. If we have children, they may be grown or nearly grown. While still working, we are less likely to see ourselves as building our career, and may imagine a day when we will cut back or even retire. Our daily lives are less structured by social institutions or socially sanctioned projects. What now?

Interestingly, our culture doesn't tell us what we are supposed to do next. Perhaps this is because people live so much longer (nearly twice as long, on average) as they did one hundred years ago; maybe our culture hasn't had time to figure out the "social clock projects" for the 60–80 age group. Perhaps it is because we are such an ageist culture that, as a society, we think it isn't important what people do at this age. Or perhaps our youth-oriented cultural outlook makes it very difficult to imagine the priorities of people who are no longer captivated by programs of outward action, material productivity, or paid work. In any case, in the United States, at the beginning of the 21st century, it may appear that the river of life has flowed steadily along a clear channel, only to become lost in a marshland where there is no clear direction, no visible current or riverbanks to contain it.

The Hidden Structure of the Life Course: Levinson's "Seasons"

Lifespan theory would say otherwise. Levinson (1978) has offered a model that, with a little tweaking, can add clarity and perspective to our vision. Levinson divides the life course into eras, each 20 years long. His research described childhood (birth–20), early (age 20–40), and middle (age 40–60) adulthood. I would suggest that we conceptualize the age 60–80 era as late adulthood, and the years beyond 80 as old age.

Within these broad eras, Levinson sees us as passing through alternate periods of stability and evaluation/transition. The evaluation/transition times surround the decade—the "age 30 transition" for example, goes from 28–32. During these transitions, we take stock of the life structure in which we live and consider modifying it to suit us better, or (if it is a transition to a new era) to better suit our priorities in the next "season" of our life. The six years between transitions are conceptualized as periods of relative stability, when we go about the business of life within the structure we have made.

FOR OUR CLINICAL WORK

As they approach or live within late adulthood, some of our clients feel lost, bewildered, at sea. While there may be other reasons for these feelings, I have found it helpful to consider them from a lifespan developmental perspective. At its best, a diagnosis can allow us to recognize patterns, possible causes, directions for treatment. A "developmental diagnosis" can do this, too. When a client has the symptoms that warrant a developmental diagnosis, we can recognize the source of the problems and can include our understandings as we talk together.

When a woman entering (or in) late adulthood asks "what now?" she may become frightened. Compared to the "social clock projects," new endeavors may seem trivial, less than. Unless we continue to do what we did when we were younger, and with the same attitude and involvement, we may fear becoming, or being seen as, "old." And yet we may not want to raise more children or try to climb higher on our career ladder.

However, if we (and our clients) begin to legitimate the five eras of life, we have a way of understanding one reason we may no longer feel "at home" in an outmoded life structure. Because each era is distinct, we allow ourselves to recognize that priorities, approaches, pleasures and burdens, preferences and concerns, will also be distinct. No era of life is about trying to continue being as you were in the era before, though there will of course be continuities and lifelong threads of interests and tastes and loves.

We can assume that we all weave predictably in and out of periods of stability and transition. Even when these are not driven by societally sanctioned momentum or the rolling of the family cycle, we (and our clients) can expect that periods of immersion will alternate with periods when we take perspective, make adjustments, try something new or renew something that had been set aside.

JULIE: TRYING TO FIND HER WAY

Julie,[1] aged 58, had always wanted to be a full-time homemaker, and she has been. After graduating college and working for a few years, she married her high school sweetheart. They have two children, now age 21 and 25. She is completing a lengthy and generally amicable divorce from her husband, who lives nearby. Julie came back to therapy (I'd seen her when her youngest was an infant) because she was angry, depressed, and felt that she was being pushed into being "a member of a group I never wanted to belong to."

The "empty nest" would have been enough of a transition for Julie. But, even though she and her husband had become very distant, the idea of having a lifelong marriage was central to Julie's expectations, to the life structure in which she saw herself. In addition, although the divorce settlement left her with sufficient money on which to live, Julie was gripped with fear about financial insecurity.

Within the essential empathic fabric of the therapy, I began to include some developmental ideas in our work. I'd mention that she was approaching a new life era, 60–80, that would be structured differently than before. We began to explore what she would want to keep, and to change, in addition to what she had to change. With the idea that all people enter a new era of life and that every life requires periods of stocktaking and modification, she gradually moved away from her view of self as victim and became more able to accept and, at times, enthusiastically engage this developmental challenge.

As she began to consider the elements that her new era's structure might have, Julie looked afresh at her enduring and loyal friendships.

---

[1]Names and potentially identifying information have been changed in the presentation of case material.

In correspondence with age mates, she began to claim and value this moment in their lives. She recalled some of the pleasures she had put aside for the demands of parenting (one was a special needs child), including a passion for designing sculptural constructions from "found objects." She continues to enjoy the times when the children come home for visits and do some of their favorite things, but she no longer "lives for those times." She has also come to recognize that her home represents and expresses who she is and can acknowledge the pleasure and satisfaction she feels living within it. A recent dissertation (Thompson, 2009) found that this aspect of one's home is psychologically central for many late adult women.

Julie has built the foundation for a life structure that provides her with vitality, self-esteem, creativity, and intimacy. Her view of herself, her expectations of how others view her, and her attitude toward living have shifted. From this foundation, there is hope that she can feel worthy to explore possibilities.

In addition to the usual benefits of psychotherapy, Julie also got substantial benefit from learning to see herself, and her problems, from a life-span developmental perspective. Levinson's theory, which gives equal weight to each era, helped her destigmatize the necessity for change that involved her reduced involvement with the culturally valued "social clock projects" that had structured her life dreams as well as her daily experience of early and middle adulthood.

The Time of Our Lives

The Irish feminist psychologist Sheila Greene has puzzled at the failure of developmental psychology to fully embrace the recognition that, both biologically and psychologically, "life is time" (Greene, 2003, p. 133). We experience the time of our lives in past, present, and future, irreversible, and always in motion. "As biological organisms," she says, "time is central to what we are, it defines the ultimate rhythm and pattern of our life, its beginning and its end" (p. 133). However, she emphasizes that we are also psychological organisms, and our psychological relationship to time is not so straightforward. Inside our subjectivity, we say "summer is coming" or "that time has passed," as if time were moving along in one direction through space, like water in a river. In industrialized countries, we have a subjective sense of time as a resource, so we can "waste time" or can "make good use of our time."

In late adulthood, time presents a paradox. On one hand, it seems to pass more quickly for older people than for younger ones. At the same time, quality of life in the here and now becomes more important (Carstensen, 1995). We also shift our perception of time when we begin thinking about time until death (Sands, 2009; Jaques, 1965), and as this occurs, "those who know they have a limited time to live appear often to find a renewed appreciation of the present and an appreciation of the richness of life, which serves to fill their days with immediate meaning, and thus effectively slows time" (Greene, 2003, p. 136).

THERAPY AND THE RIVER OF TIME

As our clients create a life structure for late adulthood, they will build on these new premises about time, and the values of our ageist, work-oriented culture will create a tension between this new meaning of time and prevailing cultural values. Middle class values in the United States today champion self-improvement (Ostrove & Stewart, 1994) and the expectation that we are all working toward a better life in the future, progressing, getting better, acquiring more. As we build a meaningful life structure for late adulthood, it will not be easy to step out of this value system, and it may be critical that we work together with a therapist who has considered these needs from a developmental perspective.

In her challenging and delightful book *Learning to be Old: Gender, Culture and Aging*, Margaret Cruikshank (2003) presents the idea that older women in a sexist/ageist culture must *learn* to be old by challenging the implicit messages we receive. Chief among these is a mandate for late adulthood that she calls "prescribed busyness." Staying "as busy as possible" is "equated with worth and mental competence" while "lack of busyness can be equated with laziness, withdrawal from others, or lack of imagination" (p. 159). This expectation, held by ourselves as well as younger people, runs counter to "a belief that the old are intrinsically worthy or that life beyond wage earning is intrinsically good" or to "the possibility that old age has meanings not shared with mid-life" (p. 160).

What are these new meanings not shared by younger people? Cruikshank includes: repose, slowing down to enjoy leisure in individual ways, the quietness of just being, carefree self-indulgence, moving to your own rhythms, altruism, creativity and creative play, experiencing things and people with more attentiveness and care, ample free time. More than any of these, she emphasizes that late adulthood can bring an awareness of spiritual values—mindfulness, deeply internal personal growth, contemplation, radical acceptance, and transcendence.

TIA, WHEN TIME IS RUNNING OUT

Tia, age 38, came to see me because she felt adrift. She was relieved to be let go from an unsatisfying job, but at a loss to find a better one. She wanted therapy to "keep her on track." I soon discovered that this "track" included a loving relationship to her partner, who had a degenerative, terminal illness. Her arrival at therapy coincided with her partner's entry into the first age (48) of a "window" of ages—from 48–55—when people die from this disease. While not chronologically inside late adulthood, Tia's partner was quite far inside the "last third of life," and many of the developmental needs of the late adult era had become important.

Accompanying a client through anticipatory grief and loss is poignant and powerful work. At the same time, keeping Tia "on track" has been very much about the ways she can approach living and their remaining time together. Central to this work has been my capacity to recognize these partners' differences in subjective time, and Tia's movement between an empathic connection to her partner's subjective time and also an awareness of her own, 38-year-old, young-to-middle-adulthood sense of her life time.

WHAT DEVELOPS DURING "ADULT DEVELOPMENT"?

Across the years of our adult lives, we all change and also, in some ways, stay the same. Certainly, some people grow more than others. I want to put words to three dimensions of psychological development in the adult years that may, if we are fortunate, invigorate and deepen the last third of life. I believe that, as therapists, we can notice and nurture these. We are accustomed to seeing ourselves as change agents and caregivers but may not have brought these developmental dimensions into focus. After describing these three dimensions, I will describe one client's integration of this developmental work.

The Development of an Ethic of Care

As theorists recognized the centrality of relationships for psychological growth, Carol Gilligan (1982) created a three-stage model for women's development. She proposed that women have a view of maturity founded on an ethic of care and that they move toward maturity through "major transitions...[that] involve changes in the understanding and activities of care" (Gilligan, 1982, p. 171).

In her three-stage model, the first stage is a focus on "caring for the self in order to ensure survival" (1982, p. 74); here, the good is identified with what serves her self-interest. This is followed by a stage in which the good is equated with a conventional view of taking responsibility and caring for others. During this stage, there is a danger that responsible care will become confused with self-sacrifice and a woman may be left unaware of her own needs and agency. As she moves toward the third stage, she begins to feel the "illogic" of the inequality between the other and the self" (p. 74) and to transcend the dilemma of selfishness versus selflessness. At this stage, she takes into account both the possibilities and limits of intervening in the lives of others as well as her responsibility for self-development (Helson, Mitchell, & Hart, 1985).

Many women seek psychotherapy because they have difficulty making their way along the early parts of this developmental trajectory. For example, the step out of self-care can be difficult for women who emerge from a childhood in which caregivers had poor boundaries or were themselves unavailable to provide responsive care for a daughter. These women are painfully challenged in couple relationships, as parents, and when asked to be collaborative with colleagues at work.

The transition from the second to the third stage may be even more challenging. As therapists, we know that—beyond urging good nutrition and daily exercise—the culture does little to describe and support self-care. We also know that women, far more than men, assume the role of primary parent of children and primary caregiver of elders (Kuchner, 1999). For many women, these are experiences of profound importance and value, and central to their sense of identity. Other women may be drawn to extraordinary levels of caring responsibility in the workplace. Whether because children grow up and elders die, or because of some growing needs of their own, many women reach a time when they want, or need, to include the self within the circle of care but struggle mightily to accomplish this in a wholehearted and unconflicted way.

Gilligan talks about women being struck by the "illogic of the inequality between self and other" (p. 74). Therapists can aid this recognition. In the face of strong, gendered cultural pressures to maintain a conventional caring stance we can help clients to ask themselves about why they do not see themselves as worthy of their care. It is a powerful moment in a psychotherapy, when a client encounters her past "illogic." A new view of self takes shape, a new self-regard. Similarly, as a woman allows herself to formulate a more differentiated understanding of the ethic of care, she recognizes the importance of blending care with the ability to let others handle their own care. A changed view of others, and of relationship, may emerge.

The Development of Integrity

In one of the first models of lifespan development, Erikson (1963) posited that the life course could be described as a sequence of eight stages. Each stage was characterized by engagement with a particular dialectic, between trust and mistrust, for example. Successful resolution of each stage involved the development of a particular psychological structure, trait, or capacity— trust, autonomy, initiative, industry (in childhood), identity and intimacy (in early adulthood), generativity (in middle adulthood), and integrity (in late adulthood).[2] While each of these dimensions continues to develop throughout life, Erikson believed that "the spotlight" of psychic energy and social circumstance focused on specific concerns at different points in the life course.

By ego integrity, the psychic integration of the final stage, Erikson (1963) was pointing to a deep sense of order, meaning the "acceptance of one's one

---

[2]Franz and White (1985) have challenged Erikson's failure to adequately describe women's development and to address the development of relational strengths in childhood. They suggest modifying the theory to create a two-path model in place of the eight individual stages so that we can chart milestones in the development of both attachment and individuation. To complement existing stages 2–5 in childhood and adolescence, they would add the development of object and self-constancy, playfulness, empathy and collaboration, and mutuality and interdependence.

and only life" (p. 268), a "comradeship with the ordering ways of distant times" (p. 268), a recognition that "an individual life is the accidental coincidence of but one life cycle with but one segment of history" (p. 268), an "emotional integration" and a "final consolidation (where) death loses its sting" (p. 268).

The stage of Integrity versus Despair has sometimes been seen as focused on a person's last days, when they look back and make a critical summation of all that came before. I disagree. Instead, I have seen that efforts to successfully resolve this dialectic are implicated in the most profound psychological undertakings of people over 60.

At the entrance to late adulthood, Erikson's theory would predict that people are concentrating on generativity (versus stagnation). We are caring for those who will live after we are gone, either by nurturing the young, conserving what is valued in our world, or creating new and useful or beautiful things that will endure to benefit future generations. As we consider the legacy we leave, we may feel some sense of generational pride—ours was the generation of the counterculture, of civil rights, feminism, gay rights. Our generation saw the birth of the computer, of genuine reproductive choices, of global citizenship, of ecological awareness. When we lay claim to the accomplishments of our "segment of history" we take a step toward that embracing of our place and time that is a cornerstone of integrity.

Even as we care for those coming up, we recognize that we must "pass the baton" to them as they run the next leg of the relay of life. This step, a central task of late adulthood, is developmentally complex. We nurture those to come not only by caring for them but also by entrusting them with responsibility (sometimes with the responsibility of caring for us). Through our willingness to give over control to future generations, we also manifest our comradeship with other times and our trust in a vast sense of order and meaning. In these ways, we transition from a focus on generativity to a manifestation of our sense of integrity.

In the task of integrity, we must lay claim to our own life, to our moment in historical time and place, with a radical acceptance: this is what has been. As elders, we take our place in the flow of life, remembering those who came before (see Flores, 2009; Bermann, 2009) and bequeathing (we hope) the best of the world we have made and maintained to those who will follow.

As we linger in the awareness that our lives will end, we may encounter the intense immediate appreciation of our world (described by Greene, 2003). These moments of appreciation, and the spiritual sub-text that surrounds them, are also ways that we express our sense of integrity.

But these accomplishments rarely come easy. With a literal "deadline" before them, women seeking psychotherapy during the last third of life may—even unconsciously—feel the urgency of these developmental steps. Our clinical work can deepen in unexpected ways when we engage our clients' needs for the development and evolution of generativity and integrity. We will want to recognize these needs as they emerge, either consciously or beneath the surface, either explicitly or represented in what they are doing, failing to do, and choosing not to do. We, as psychotherapists, can hope to be ready, to be able to detect these concerns and address them.

To be ready, though, we may have our own personal work to do. We will need to find a way to metabolize our personal narcissism enough to deeply accept our own death and the smallness of our lives in the vastness of the river of life and time (see Loeb, 2009). Only then can we meet these concerns in our clients with the comfort, understanding, and containment they have come to expect from our psychotherapy relationship.

The Development of a Mature Ego

In psychodynamic theory, the ego is the structure within the psyche that synthesizes the contributions of every part. Ego development, then, is akin to individuation or the development of the self. When Jane Loevinger (1976) says that the ego develops, she is talking about systematic changes in style of life, method of facing problems, opinions about self and others, character, cognitive style, interpersonal relations, impulse control, conscious preoccupations, and moral judgment.

Loevinger's theory describes the ego's development as passage through a series of stages. While there are five stages in her theory, research on thousands of adults has shown that most people stop just beyond the second of these five. A mature, well-developed ego is rare and often hard won.

How do people at the various stages differ? Briefly, the first, "self-protective" stage is characterized by cognitive simplicity, a manipulative interpersonal style, a preoccupation with control, and a desire to protect oneself. One fears being caught and externalizes blame. A desire to belong, to be "normal" and "happy," to fill one's role, and a preoccupation with appearance and acceptability are keynotes of the second, conformist, stage.

At the third stage, a person has moved beyond simple self-protection and a focus on belonging. A sense of choice emerges, and the self is seen as the origin of one's destiny. Inwardly, a person lives more by self-evaluated standards and pays attention to patterns, motives, ideals, and concerns for self-respect. Interpersonally, communication becomes very important as the superficial is replaced by a desire for authentic mutuality.

In the fourth and fifth stages, the individual lives in an internal atmosphere of psychic autonomy. There is an acceptance of inner conflict and internal locus of control. Self-fulfillment emerges as a personal goal. There is a growing awareness of emotional interdependence, a pleasuring in this facet of human experience, and a cherishing both of individuality and of personal ties. An increasing objectivity develops along with a capacity to see from multiple perspectives. Fear of the unknown is rare; instead, openness to the future and tolerance for ambiguity characterize this ego stage. Cognitive style is increasingly complex, tolerant of ambiguity and contradiction, and conscious preoccupations are less superficial and concrete. Emotions are differentiated and vividly conveyed (Helson et al., 1985).

As therapists, we recognize that many characteristics of a mature, developed ego may equally describe the kind of psychological maturity that we wish for our clients and for ourselves. Much about psychotherapy is already in the service of encouraging and consolidating ego development. How does the ego develop? Loevinger says that new structure comes about when we cannot fully take in and work on what is happening by using the intrapsychic structure we have. Our current "tool kit" isn't adequate; something more is needed.

In the relational field of therapy, new material comes into view. Sometimes we need, and acquire, new tools, new psychological structure, to allow this material into our consciousness. In addition to our usual ways of accomplishing this, we therapists can sensitize ourselves to particular ego challenges and become able to recognize them as part of a developmental process. When we put this process into words, this may expand our client's access to the strengths needed to complete these changes.

An Example of Developmental Work in Therapy

I met Betty, aged 60, four months after she had to leave work and go on disability. Initially, an infection required bed rest. But once in bed, she found herself unable to concentrate on anything; it took more than three tries to read a newspaper article. Her partner and teenaged child took care of her, frightened and astonished by the change in a woman who had been a dynamo.

These symptoms had abated somewhat before she came to see me. Betty said that she had "heard the wakeup call" but she was terrified that she would somehow drift back into her old way of doing things, a way that could easily have led to her premature death.

How had she created a life of endless demands? As a child, she had admired her parents' success in the community and aspired to match their commitment to service. As an adult, this translated into training for a helping profession, where her talents and availability led to her steady advancement. She was an outstanding and caring team leader of an ever-expanding team that eventually spanned several states.

With minimal opportunity or motivation to focus on herself, she had paid no attention to her health or to any need for solitude, relaxation, fun, creativity, intimacy. By the time she contracted the infection, she was entirely depleted, and friends and family had learned to expect nothing from her.

A NEW ERA OF LIFE, AND A NEW LIFE STRUCTURE

As Betty and I sat together with her fears and her bewilderment, I recognized that this health crisis had resulted, in part, from Betty's inability to notice that she was no longer thriving; the life structure she had made no longer suited her. As she told me about her life, it became clear that her early identifications and values had made it almost unthinkable for Betty to consider stepping back and evaluating her service-dominated structure.

Learning that, at 60, she was stepping into a new era of life, was a great relief to Betty. It lifted her fear that she must choose between saving herself and betraying her values. It also allowed her to approach the next "chapter" in her life rather than feel stalled in a sense of failure at being unable to continue as she had been. She started stocktaking in earnest: what about her life no longer worked, no longer suited her? What might she want instead? What did she want for the coming 20-year era?

She did not want to work all the time. In fact, one thing that she wanted was to have time—both longevity and a daily dose of unscheduled time for her personal use. She decided that, once she got a medical okay to return to work, she would return as a "frontline" service provider and leave administration with its endless demands behind.

Once she could see her new life without self-blame or feelings of guilt, the unscheduled days required for her continuing medical recovery provided her the opportunity to consider what (besides work) she enjoyed. She read, kept a journal, began taking walks, started puttering in her backyard. As her health improved, family time was important, and she had energy for bedtime talks with her partner.

INCLUDING HERSELF IN THE ETHIC OF CARE

Betty and I paid a lot of attention to her child's-eye view of her parents as models of caregiving. Through this careful history, Betty began to think about care, caregiving over time, how she had diminished her family-related caregiving in response to work demands. Her physician had required a regimen of self-care, and as we talked about how strange and new it felt, Betty began to consider why she felt so odd when she took care of herself and so comfortable taking charge of others' care.

As this material emerged into consciousness, a day came when, as Gilligan would have predicted, the "illogic of the inequality of self and other" lit up. In that moment, possibly for the first time since childhood, Betty was able to approach herself with compassion, kindness, understanding—all of the tender qualities she had directed toward others. Inside this experience, she took in the emotion of both giving this care and of receiving it. Now that this was possible, she saw herself differently. Her understanding of care had broadened.

THE TIME OF HER LIFE

Betty had been badly frightened by this health crisis. Now she knew, as never before, that she wasn't able to "withstand more than most people." Like the rest of us, she was only human, with all of the vulnerability that comes with it. Most of her relatives had long lives, and she expected to have many more years. Now, she'd become aware of the possibility of her own death, and this catapulted her into a very different way of looking at time.

Betty described the intense immediate appreciation of life associated with knowing it will end soon. She would come to a therapy session and talk about the glories of the weather, the feeling of the air on her skin, or a bird in the backyard. She was not very interested in long-range plans but very engaged in making plans for her partner's birthday or taking a weekend trip. Consistent with this view, she began reading books by an author on Oprah's list (Echkhard Tolle) who advocates living "in the now," and she used these to encourage herself to cultivate her new perspective on time.

THE EVOLUTION OF GENERATIVITY AND DEVELOPMENT OF INTEGRITY

When she returned to work, Betty was surprised that supervisory, leadership, and administrative tasks kept presenting themselves, despite her explicit request to provide only direct service. She began planning ways that she could gently decline, and as she did so she became aware that she was putting words to her new recognition that her colleagues "would find their own way" and "it was theirs to do now."

Similarly, Betty recognized this same stepping back when her older child came home from college for a visit. Her nurturance took a new form: appreciating his independence and his capacity to do things around the house. He had his own life now, and this led her to think about her own life. She mused about the differences in the world he was entering and the one she stepped into as a young adult. Gradually, she became more conscious of her place in history, her style. She liked her life, so different from his.

BETTY'S EGO MATURES

As our work continued, I noticed that much had changed about the kinds of conversations that Betty and I were having. In the early part of our work, she was frightened, overwhelmed, bewildered. She had held herself to some simple ideas about how a person should live, and life had brought her new experiences that she had no way to understand. As a result, she had to find new ways of looking at herself and her life, new ways of thinking about it. This is the very process that catalyzes ego development.

Without using psychological jargon, I would describe Betty's predicament to her, putting words to her developmental needs and gently suggesting that perhaps she could allow herself to try some new approaches, that perhaps she was capable of generating these new perspectives.

She was, indeed. Her changes match closely to the way a more mature ego functions. Betty has become very interested in her personal growth, taken up meditation, and begun an interest in Eastern philosophies. Though she returned to work, she is not much interested in talking about it; instead, she looks forward to telling me about the end of her workday when she walks home, clears her mind, and has a few hours of solitude before the other family members come home. She has gotten interested in her own inner life. Her thinking seems to be richer, more multifaceted and complex than before. After years of giving little attention to friends and family, she is delighted to get to know them anew. Her perceptions and emotions are vivid and clear. She is curious about what's coming next and doesn't need to take charge of it.

CONCLUSION

I have focused on a few of the many lifespan developmental models and concepts that can inform our personal psychological work and our psychotherapy in the last third of life. These are ways that academic psychology can influence what we do. But the direction of influence could go the other way as well. One way of looking at our psychotherapy work is that we are always researchers, doing experiments with one or two people at a time. In academic psychology, these are called N = 1 studies, and they have taught us much about the workings of the psyche.

Whether out of ageism or because it's so new for humans to live so long, psychologists have theorized, named, understood relatively little about this third of the human lifespan. Psychotherapists, with their many N = 1 studies, have the potential to make a great contribution to our knowledge. In this area, we can move toward closing the embrace of the two arms of psychology, bringing together the academic and the clinical—completing a circle— a gesture that is a hallmark of this developmental period.

REFERENCES

Bermann, A. (2009). Reflections on aging, psychotherapy, and spiritual practice. *Women and Therapy, 33*(2–4).

Carstensen, L. (1995). Evidence for a lifespan theory of socio-emotional selectivity. *Current Directions in Psychological Science, 4*, 151–156.

Cruikshank, M. (2003). *Learning to be old: Gender, culture and aging.* Lanham, MD: Rowman and Littlefield Publishers.

Erikson, E. (1963). *Childhood and society.* New York: Norton.

Flores, Y. (2009). On becoming an elder: An immigrant Latina therapist narrative. *Women and Therapy, 33*(2–4).

Franz, C., & White, K. (1985). Indiviuation and attachment in personality development: Extending Erikson's theory. *Journal of Personality, 53*, 224–256.

Gilligan, C. (1982). *In a different voice: Psychological theory and women's development.* Cambridge, MA: Harvard University Press.

Greene, S. (2003). *The psychological development of girls and women: Rethinking Change in time*. New York: Routledge.

Helson, R., Mitchell, V., & Hart, B. (1985). Lives of women who became autonomous. *Journal of Personality, 53*, 257–285.

Helson, R., Mitchell, V., & Moane, G. (1984). Personality and patterns of adherence and non-adherence to the social clock. *Journal of Personality and Social Psychology, 46*, 1079–1096.

Jaques, E. (1965). Death and the mid-life crisis. *International Journal of Psychoanalysis, 46*, 502–514.

Kuchner, J. (1999). The sandwich generation: Women's roles as multi-generational caregivers. In C. Forden, A. Hunter, & B. Birns (Eds.), *Readings in the psychology of women: Dimensions of the female experience* (pp. 231–241). Boston, MA: Allyn & Bacon.

Levinson, D. J. (1978). *Seasons of a man's life*. New York: Knopf.

Loeb, E. (2009). The therapist at 60, the patient at 60: Challenges for psychotherapy. *Women and Therapy, 33*(2–4).

Loevinger, J. (1976). *Ego development: Conceptions and theories*. San Francisco, CA: Jossey-Bass.

Ostrove, J., & Stewart, A. (1994). Meanings and uses of marginal identities: Social class at Radcliffe in the 1960s. In C. Franz & A. Stewart (Eds.), *Women creating lives: Identifies, resilience and resistance* (pp. 289–308). Boulder, CO: Westview Press.

Sands, S. (2009). Less time ahead, more behind: Being a psychotherapist in the last third of life. *Women and Therapy, 33*(2–4).

Thompson, M. (2009). The home as an expression of the self. Unpublished doctoral dissertation, California School of Professional Psychology at Alliant University, San Francisco, California.

Index